Progressing Critical Posthuman Perspectives in Health Sociology

This book shows the potential of posthuman thinking for rethinking healthcare, experiences, subjects and interventions. It explores a range of posthuman dilemmas across diverse health issues as contributors grapple with the ethical, ontological and epistemological relations of knowing and doing health.

The volume problematises the rational, agentic individual as the key driver of health-related action and experience. Contributors move beyond long-held humanist assumptions about health, illness, and well-being, and attune – theoretically and methodologically – to the entangled relations or ecologies that instantiate realities. They reimagine how care practices and healthcare experiences materialise through human-non-human relationality as biosocial environments. Chapters explore and articulate the agency of more-than-human entities in health-related processes to shed new light on health interventions, evaluations and health policy. Taken together, the book highlights that although posthumanism enables health sociologists to progress particular agendas, it is essential to further problematise the posthuman decentring of the human by bringing sustained attention to bear on the ethical and political implications of this approach to knowledge-making in health. This field-defining collection consolidates and builds momentum in the burgeoning area of posthuman thinking in health.

It will appeal to scholars and researchers seeking to understand health as a relational achievement better. This book was originally published as a special issue of *Health Sociology Review*.

Kim McLeod is Senior Lecturer in Sociology at the School of Social Sciences at the University of Tasmania, Tasmania, Australia. Kim re-envisions health and education in her academic work towards equitable access, experiences and outcomes.

Simone Fullagar is Professor and Chair of the Sport and Gender Equity research hub and Lead for the Inclusive Play theme in the Reimagining Disability research programme at Griffith University, Queensland, Australia. Simone is an interdisciplinary sociologist who undertakes research to address gender inequality in sport, leisure, mental health and well-being as more-than-human issues.

Progressing Critical Posthuman Perspectives in Health Sociology

Edited by
Kim McLeod and Simone Fullagar

Routledge
Taylor & Francis Group
LONDON AND NEW YORK

First published 2025
by Routledge
2 Park Square, Milton Park, Abingdon, Oxon OX14 4RN

and by Routledge
52 Vanderbilt Avenue, New York, NY 10017

Routledge is an imprint of the Taylor & Francis Group, an informa business

British Library Cataloguing in Publication Data
A catalogue record for this book is available from the British Library

ISBN13: 978-1-032-81249-6
ISBN13: 978-1-032-81252-6
ISBN13: 978-1-003-49889-6

DOI: 10.4324/9781003498896

Typeset in Minion Pro
by Newgen Publishing UK

Publisher's Note
The publisher accepts responsibility for any inconsistencies that may have arisen during the conversion of this book from journal articles to book chapters, namely the inclusion of journal terminology.

Contents

Citation Information vi
Notes on Contributors viii

Introduction – Remaking the post 'human': a productive problem for health sociology 1
Kim McLeod and Simone Fullagar

1 Becoming posthuman: hepatitis C, the race to elimination and the politics of remaking the subject 11
Kate Seear and Emily Lenton

2 Making publics in a pandemic: Posthuman relationalities, 'viral' intimacies and COVID-19 26
Kiran Pienaar, Jacinthe Flore, Jennifer Power and Dean Murphy

3 Domestic violence, coercive control and mental health in a pandemic: disenthralling the ecology of the domestic 42
Toni McCallum and Judy Rose

4 Lost in translation? Beyond sex as a biological variable in animal research 57
Madeleine Pape

5 A posthuman decentring of person-centred care 74
Barbara E. Gibson, Joanna K. Fadyl, Gareth Terry, Kate Waterworth, Donya Mosleh and Nicola M. Kayes

6 Materialities of care for older people: caring together/apart in the political economy of caring apparatus 90
Michela Cozza, Silvia Bruzzone and Lucia Crevani

7 Afflexivity in post-qualitative inquiry: prioritising affect and reflexivity in the evaluation of a health information website 105
Jenny Setchell, Rebecca Olson, Merrill Turpin, Nathalia Costa, Tim Barlott, Kate O'Halloran, Britta Wigginton and Paul Hodges

Index 121

Citation Information

The chapters in this book were originally published in the *Health Sociology Review*, volume 30, issue 3 (2021). When citing this material, please use the original page numbering for each article, as follows:

Introduction

Remaking the post 'human': a productive problem for health sociology
Kim McLeod and Simone Fullagar
Health Sociology Review, volume 30, issue 3 (2021), pp. 219–228

Chapter 1

Becoming posthuman: hepatitis C, the race to elimination and the politics of remaking the subject
Kate Seear and Emily Lenton
Health Sociology Review, volume 30, issue 3 (2021), pp. 229–243

Chapter 2

Making publics in a pandemic: Posthuman relationalities, 'viral' intimacies and COVID-19
Kiran Pienaar, Jacinthe Flore, Jennifer Power and Dean Murphy
Health Sociology Review, volume 30, issue 3 (2021), pp. 244–259

Chapter 3

Domestic violence, coercive control and mental health in a pandemic: disenthralling the ecology of the domestic
Toni McCallum and Judy Rose
Health Sociology Review, volume 30, issue 3 (2021), pp. 260–274

Chapter 4

Lost in translation? Beyond sex as a biological variable in animal research
Madeleine Pape
Health Sociology Review, volume 30, issue 3 (2021), pp. 275–291

Chapter 5

A posthuman decentring of person-centred care
Barbara E. Gibson, Joanna K. Fadyl, Gareth Terry, Kate Waterworth, Donya Mosleh and Nicola M. Kayes
Health Sociology Review, volume 30, issue 3 (2021), pp. 292–307

Chapter 6

Materialities of care for older people: caring together/apart in the political economy of caring apparatus
Michela Cozza, Silvia Bruzzone and Lucia Crevani
Health Sociology Review, volume 30, issue 3 (2021), pp. 308–322

Chapter 7

Afflexivity in post-qualitative inquiry: prioritising affect and reflexivity in the evaluation of a health information website
Jenny Setchell, Rebecca Olson, Merrill Turpin, Nathalia Costa, Tim Barlott, Kate O'Halloran, Britta Wigginton and Paul Hodges
Health Sociology Review, volume 30, issue 3 (2021), pp. 323–338

Notes on Contributors

Tim Barlott, Faculty of Rehabilitation Medicine, University of Alberta, Alberta, Canada.

Silvia Bruzzone, Department of Organization and Management, Mälardalen University, Västerås, Sweden.

Nathalia Costa, School of Health and Rehabilitation Sciences, The University of Queensland, Brisbane, Australia.

Michela Cozza, Department of Organization and Management, Mälardalen University, Västerås, Sweden.

Lucia Crevani, Department of Organization and Management, Mälardalen University, Västerås, Sweden.

Joanna K. Fadyl, Centre for Person Centred Research, Auckland University of Technology, Auckland, New Zealand.

Jacinthe Flore, Historical and Philosophical Studies, University of Melbourne, Melbourne, Australia.

Simone Fullagar, Centre for Social and Cultural Research, Griffith University, Queensland, Australia.

Barbara E. Gibson, Department of Physical Therapy, University of Toronto and Bloorview Research Institute, Holland Bloorview Kids Rehabilitation Hospital, Ontario, Canada.

Kate O'Halloran, National Ageing Research Institute, Melbourne, Australia.

Paul Hodges, School of Health and Rehabilitation Sciences, The University of Queensland, Brisbane, Australia.

Nicola M. Kayes, Centre for Person Centred Research, Auckland University of Technology, Auckland, New Zealand.

Emily Lenton, Australian Research Centre in Sex, Health and Society, La Trobe University, Bundoora, Australia.

Toni McCallum, Indigenous Futures, Education & Arts, Charles Darwin University, Darwin, Australia.

Kim McLeod, School of Social Sciences, University of Tasmania, Tasmania, Australia.

Donya Mosleh, Rehabilitation Sciences Institute, University of Toronto, Ontario, Canada.

Dean Murphy, Kirby Institute, University of New South Wales, Sydney, Australia.

Rebecca Olson, School of Social Science, The University of Queensland, Brisbane, Australia.

Madeleine Pape, Institute of Sports Sciences, University of Lausanne, Lausanne, Switzerland.

Kiran Pienaar, School of Humanities and Social Sciences, Deakin University, Melbourne, Australia; School of Social Sciences, Monash University, Melbourne, Australia.

Jennifer Power, Australian Research Centre for Sex, Health and Society (ARCSHS), La Trobe University, Melbourne, Australia.

Judy Rose, Faculty of Arts, Education and Law, Griffith University, Brisbane, Australia.

Kate Seear, Australian Research Centre in Sex, Health and Society, La Trobe University, Bundoora, Australia.

Jenny Setchell, Institute for Urban Indigenous Health, Brisbane, Australia.

Gareth Terry, Centre for Person Centred Research, Auckland University of Technology, Auckland, New Zealand.

Merrill Turpin, School of Health and Rehabilitation Sciences, The University of Queensland, Brisbane, Australia.

Kate Waterworth, Centre for Person Centred Research, Auckland University of Technology, Auckland, New Zealand.

Britta Wigginton, School of Public Health, The University of Queensland, Brisbane, Australia.

[illegible]

[illegible]

[illegible]

[illegible]

[illegible]

[illegible]

[illegible]

[illegible]

[illegible]

[illegible]

[illegible]

[illegible]

[illegible]

[illegible]

Introduction – Remaking the post 'human': a productive problem for health sociology

Kim McLeod and Simone Fullagar

We start by acknowledging we are writing on the unceded lands of the palawa and pakana peoples of lutrawita (Tasmania), and the Yugambeh and Kombumerri peoples. This is important because contemporary sociological paradigms such as posthumanism, the subject of this editorial, sometimes overlook how the politics of colonisation continues to shape academic knowledge production (which this editorial goes on to discuss).

The figure of the post 'human' is entangled in a set of dilemmas that are useful for informing sociological ways of thinking through health matters in more than human worlds. The complexities of living in a COVID society (Lupton & Willis, 2021; Matthewman & Huppatz, 2020), the challenges of climate change and persistent inequalities all emphasise the need to better understand the material and discursive forces shaping the conditions of health for people who exist in a dynamic relation with the planet. Posthuman approaches are generative here, making visible the more than human forces and power relations that constitute subjectivity and health practices (Fox & Alldred, 2016; Pyyhtinen, 2016; Willcox, Hickey-Moody, & Harris, 2021). Moving beyond the sociological parameters of social structure and human agency, posthumanism challenges us to engage more deeply with the onto-ethical-epistemological assumptions that inform all research approaches (Barad, 2007). Troubling long-held humanist assumptions about health, illness and wellbeing also calls for sociologists to attune – theoretically and methodologically - to the entangled relations or ecologies that instantiate realities. The articles in this special issue explore a range of posthuman dilemmas across diverse health issues as they grapple with the ethical, ontological and epistemological relations of knowing and doing health.

In this editorial, we discuss how the papers in this special issue harness posthuman approaches to further a range of productive lines of enquiry and knowledge-making for health sociology. Using posthuman perspectives enables the authors to generate health sociology knowledge beyond humanist assumptions, ideals and logics and rethink health care, experiences, subjects and interventions. We go on to argue that although posthumanism enables health sociologists to progress particular agendas, it is important to further problematise the posthuman decentring of the human by bringing sustained attention to bear on the ethical and political implications of this approach to knowledge-making in health. In the latter half of this editorial, we explore three strategies for responding to the limitations, gaps and silences in posthuman thinking about health that have been inspired by Indigenous, decolonial and feminist scholars with respect to unlearning Western privilege (traditions, logics and notions of selfhood, etc). The strategies include orientating to posthuman thinking as a provincial (Meghji, 2021; Mignolo & Walsh, 2018), pluriversal (Blaser & de la Cadena, 2018; Mignolo, 2000), and situated (Moreton-Robinson, 2013; Todd, 2016) endeavour. We suggest these strategies facilitate critical questioning about remaking the post 'human' in relation to the assumptions and practices that shape sociological research processes. Approaching the post 'human' as a productive problem is a means to progress the conversation between health sociology and posthumanism.

Using the 'remade' human to progress health sociology

The papers in the special issue contribute to the experiment happening in health sociology with what Seear and Lenton (2021) describe in this special issue as the 'remade' human and exemplify how taking up the 'remade' human generates a range of productive lines of enquiry and knowledge-making for health sociology. A key tenant of posthuman perspectives is to problematise the rational, agentic individual as the key driver of action and experience. Instead, posthuman frameworks propose that socio-material practices and processes produce the human as a relational achievement. As Alaimo (2017) suggests this is a question concerning 'how bodies, substances, technologies, and environments not only are acted upon but also act. Matter is not inert but instead is active, lively, and sometimes surprising' (p. xv).

Cozza, Bruzzone, and Crevani (2021) and Gibson et al. (2021) explore how care practices and experiences of healthcare materialise through human-non-human relationality as biosocial environments. These papers show how different ways of thinking about health care are enabled if care is thought of as an entanglement of materialities and the cared-for person is enacted through clinical and care arrangements. Care is figured as a material<>discursive relation that becomes enacted through the affective forces of health assemblages involving human habits, nonhuman objects, systems of classification, surfaces, organisational knowledges and flows of capital (de La Bellacasa, 2017). This approach brings into focus the relations that are embedded in ways of thinking and doing care, patienthood, illness and health without presuming a pre-existing, agentic individual as the starting point. The paper by Gibson et al. (2021) provides a compelling example of how patient-centred care can be rethought beyond humanist assumptions to open up ethical responses to 'person-care' as a dynamic assemblage. Informed by healthcare scholarship that draws together science and technology studies, disability studies and the sociology of health their posthumanist perspective enacts an 'epistemic activism' to contest the territorialisation of modes of care (for others, rather than with others) within health services. In this way, the articulation of new ways of practicing, organising and enacting health care *with* people with disability – as a process of becoming rather than static classification – can invite conversation with existing ways of knowing and doing (limitations and possibilities). Thinking with these assemblage formations of health care can work to make intelligible the normalised and the novel care processes through which subjectivities materialise in particular ways. By troubling the relations of force that circulate through expert and lay knowledges, researcher-practitioner-patient relations can create emergent spaces for different voices, bodies and desires.

The authors in the special issue take up a key feature of posthuman thinking in relation to health-related issues and questions. They explore and articulate the agency of more-than-human entities in health-related processes to shed new light on health interventions, evaluations and health policy (Vitellone, 2017). This approach enables Setchell et al. (2021) to switch the conventional direction of activity and ask, how a material website about managing back pain interacts with humans. They show how the assembling in relation to the website both makes an impression, and does not attend to complexities of back management. Setchell et al. (2021) invite us to rethink what is included in health evaluation strategies. Pienaar, Flore, Power, and Murphy (2021) also identify and challenge the norms of kinship, relationship and sexuality that are co-produced with the human subject enacted by Covid-19 public health advice. Setchell et al. (2021) and Pienaar et al. (2021) demonstrate how posthuman perspectives enable investigation into how health is mediated in the affective and embodied registers of experience (Coffey, 2020). This is an important perspective to advance discussion beyond couching health interventions as purely representational matters.

To attend to socio-material practices and processes of assembling, provokes questions about the ethical stance taken by researchers. Authors in this special issue, and across health sociology more broadly, draw on Barad's (2007, 2012) notion of 'response-ability'. They bring an ethical mode of attention to how realities and worlds are produced via posthuman research processes and cultivate capacity for response (McLeod, 2014a). Gibson et al. (2021) consider the ethics of care, and formulate care as in-the-moment recognition of the productive potential to do differently (p. 12). Pape (2021) also asks, what kind of response-abilities might sociologists develop to better engage with the nonhuman dimensions of knowledge projects, particularly as they relate to health, difference and other truth claims? The lines of enquiry enabled by such ethical stances are linked with political intent. For example, they have been shown to further participatory harm reduction praxis in alcohol and other drugs sociology (Dennis & Farrugia, 2017; Duff, 2015).

Feminist, decolonial, Indigenous, ecological and more than human scholars have contributed to the growing body of work on political and ethical frameworks that are informing different posthuman thinking about health and wellbeing (Arnold, Atchison, & McKnight, 2021; Braidotti, 2020; McLeod, 2017). As Karen Barad has argued through a posthuman feminist and queer politics, questions of knowledge production (about health) are not simply about what differences exist but 'how differences get made, what gets excluded and, how those exclusions matter' (Barad, 2007, p. 20) through the 'cuts' of apparatus (methods, concepts, histories). In this sense, politics and ethics shape the kind of matter that is valued, how relations are imagined, and the kinds of communities which are evoked (Mignolo & Walsh, 2018). At stake in sociological research are ethico-onto-epistemological questions that take seriously the politics of matter and the implications for rethinking the mind-body, normal-abnormal, healthy-ill dualisms (Fullagar, 2017). As an example, critical approaches to researching the conditions shaping and alleviating 'mental ill health' importantly identify social inequalities. However, sociological insights have tended to bracket out more complex questions about how distress materialises through entangled biopsychosocial relations and practices, as well as recovery and prevention approaches (Fullagar, O'Brien, & Pavlidis, 2019). In contrast, a posthuman sociology of health can contribute to cross and transdisciplinary thinking that understands the 'social' as imbricated in knowledge practices that produce biological, ecological and technological phenomena (such as, policies, habits, objects, bodies).

The papers in the special issue bring careful attention to how difference is made (gender, sexuality, race, ability, age and animals, nature, places), and what interests and needs are included and excluded in and through the assembling processes. Conceptualising health care contexts including research and policies as socio-material, brings into view how diverse bodies can be understood as entangled phenomena. Mcallum and Rose (2021) draw upon insights from science and technology studies to their analysis of domestic violence, coercive control and mental health in a pandemic. They develop a neo-ecological framework (Hörl, 2017) to examine the socio-material practices through which coercive control is enacted. This way of thinking about home as an ecology places emphasis on *relational* processes that constitute hybridity, in particular the inter-dependencies of human and non-human actors. Through a feminist perspective they show how practices to cope with coercive control traverse and are countered through socio-material practices including bodies, spaces, time, pets, money and technologies.

Pape's (2021) article in this issue also pursues a feminist posthumanism that produces a detailed analysis of the tensions that arise when progressive intent (pursuing gender equality) meets biological reductionism (the givenness of 'sex' as a variable) in the formulation of new health policy and research. Focussing on the US National Institutes of Health policy that mandates sex as a consideration in basic and preclinical research (Sex as a Biological Variable, SABV), Pape explores how cell lines and animal models are positioned as the key to future knowledge production that is more gender equal, given the historical dominance of masculine models. What Pape's analysis shows is how nonhuman laboratory animals are recruited into biomedical researchers' enactments of sex/gender difference and how their actions also trouble universalised notions of binary difference. This sensibility towards the actions of the more-than-human enables learning from laboratory animals in ways that reveal the contextual characteristics of sex - the multiplicity and elusiveness that points to the discursive formation of 'biological' variables. In recognising this material<>discursive entanglement, Pape considers what animal models 'do' to trouble the production and translation of biological knowledge into policy that advocates for human health. In this work, we hear the echo of Barad's (2015, p. 388) queer politics that explores different possibilities for 'the nature of matter and its agential capacities for imaginative, desiring, and affectively charged forms of bodily engagements'. The uptake of posthuman thinking as exemplified by the papers in this special issue, and by health sociology more broadly, suggest the diverse forms of knowledge-making enabled by posthumanism align with and progress agendas valued by health sociology. As Seear and Lenton (2021) observe, posthuman approaches 'open up an important political space, pushing back against foundational logics of drug law, policy and related fields of practice' (p. 3). Similarly, Gibson et al. (2021) suggest that posthuman thinking enables exploration of care in addition to approaches which are 'limited by humanist ideals of choice, autonomy, and self-determination' (p. 9).

Seear and Lenton (2021) invite critical thinking about the implications of the posthuman remade human. They track how the policy and practice shifts associated with the race to eliminate Hepatitis C recompose the subject (people who live with Hep C/people who use drugs) through changing relations between people, medicine, the State, medical policy and drugs. They identify how rights and forms of care deemed valuable by the individual are erased through the recomposing, and how this constitutes a dilemma for people who live with Hep C/people who use drugs. Seear and Lenton (2021) observe this also presents a dilemma for posthuman scholarship. We suggest such a stance – bringing close examination to bear on the political consequences of the 'problem' of the remade human in their contexts, *and* how posthuman conceptual and methodological tools co-create the remade human – can progress the conversation between health sociology and posthumanism. As Seear and Lenton (2021) show, this stance focuses attention on how re-makings can be 'simultaneously homogenising, humanising and dehumanising' (p. 10). There is, we suggest, an important positive consequence of approaching posthumanism's co-construction of the remade human as a dilemma. It invites more explicit engagement with, and accounting for, the predominantly Anglo-European political and ethical frameworks which travel alongside posthuman thinking. In making a decisive break with the human, posthuman scholarship can elide the extent to which it continues to contribute towards philosophical debates about who counts as human and who does not. Scholarship in this special issue can be regarded as a jump off point to future research agendas in health that can extend the sociological imagination in new ways. We go on to discuss how entering more fully into this debate has potential to progress posthuman health sociology.

Making political and ethical commitments explicit

Accounting for how the politics of colonialism shapes posthuman thinking is an important aspect of making explicit the political and ethical frameworks which accompany posthuman thinking. Decolonial thinkers highlight how conceptions of humanity are seared to colonial practices and as a consequence colonised people are not recognised as fully human (Weheliye, 2014; Wynter, 2003; Wynter & McKittrick, 2015). Scholars draw on this insight to trouble how the move from humanist to posthumanist knowledges insufficiently acknowledges and challenges the working of modernity to reduce the majority of the population to less-than-human (Blaser & de la Cadena, 2018; Mignolo & Walsh, 2018; Zembylas, 2018). Mignolo and Walsh (2018, p. 117) unpack how the idea of a universal posthuman 'we' perpetuates a universal version of history moving through premodern, modern, postmodern and anthropocene times which has the effect of negating a pluriversality of histories. The tendency of posthuman thinking to attribute the nature/culture binary as a universal phenomenon has been widely critiqued by Indigenous and decolonial scholars who point out this represents a regional concern of western scholars: nature and culture are concepts only valid within western cosmology (Mignolo & Walsh, 2018; Todd, 2016). The politics of colonialism is also enacted in posthuman thinking via the non-recognition of Indigenous ontologies and the problem of colonising rather than validating Indigenous worldviews and ways of thinking, doing and being (Joronen & Häkli, 2017; Todd, 2016; Tuhiwai Smith, 2012).

Scholars bring a decolonial lens to critique the posthuman shifting of power away from the human and onto the distributed agency of self-organising matter. By attributing unequal power primarily to Anthropomorphism, posthuman frameworks are challenged for eliding the power linked to the colonial western gaze (Mignolo & Walsh, 2018; Schulz, 2017; Zembylas, 2018). As López (2018) explains, the move of re-inscribing all that is non-human as having thing-power effectively makes those humans not in charge of the world, legible through being vibrant matter. López' charge to posthuman thinking is: 'such a theory simply cannot explain why it does not itself function as a "racializing assemblage" in its positing of a raceless liberal humanist subject confronting "vibrant matter"' (2018, p. 383). As this brief overview of some of the decolonial critique of posthuman thinking indicates, posthuman thinking needs to account for how its theory and methods are shaped by colonisation. This points to the importance of making political and ethical commitments explicit – decolonial and Indigenous scholars suggest a range of strategies, including articulating a position in relation to the extent to which posthuman thinking is provincial, pluriversal and situated.

The first strategy is to ensure posthuman thinking is engaged with as a *provincial endeavour*. This entails defining posthuman thinking in its historical and colonial context: arising from the regional and limited concerns of Eurocentrism, with a particular interest in rejecting the human based on a critique of European humanism (Mignolo & Walsh, 2018; Todd, 2016). This perspective draws attention to the partial specificity of the theoretical framework and its 'unstated norms and assumptions' (Lawhon, Silver, Ernstson, & Pierce, 2016, p. 1619). A provincial posthuman framework destabilises a political commitment to the universal world, an abstract universal or more-than-human. It invites questions about the imaginings of relations, global community and political action enabled by the framework, thus avoiding what Meghji (2021) describes as the unreflexive reproduction of the Eurocentric perspective. Scholars who seek to progress a decolonial agenda propose a useful way to reveal how every perspective is provincial and partial: putting theoretical perspectives into conversation (Meghji, 2021). Paur (2017) exemplifies this approach, bringing intersectionality and assemblage thinking together in a way that allows for the tension between the frameworks; Zembylas (2018) puts Wynter and Braidotti together to give priority to the task of decolonisation, and open up the ethics of relational ways of being/doing. A provincial posthuman framework, which accounts for how it arises from a colonial context, is better equipped to enter into respectful conversation with Indigenous literatures and philosophies about agential realism (Rosiek, Snyder, & Pratt, 2020; Todd, 2016).

The second strategy provides further means of challenging the *universalising* gestures of posthuman thought: bringing posthuman thinking into contact with the decolonial concept of the pluriverse. The pluriverse denotes multiple co-existing worlds (Blaser & de la Cadena, 2018; Mignolo, 2000). A pluriversal view of more-than-human ontologies shifts attention from the universal onto the dynamics through which different worlds or ontologies bring themselves into being and importantly the interaction and contestation between different worlds (Mignolo & Walsh, 2018). A purposeful orientation towards the pluriverse enables questioning of eurocentrism in theory and practice (McLeod et al., 2020). Importantly, a pluriversal perspective facilitates more serious engagement with the multiplicity of lifeworlds and a commitment to deeply understand how our different understandings and experiences position ourselves in relation to each other (Schulz, 2017; Sundberg, 2014). The principle of pluriversal co-existence underpins a world 'in which the radical differences between hegemonic and Indigenous standpoints are not suppressed' (Mignolo, 2005, p. 106).

A pluriversal orientation provides posthuman health sociology with greater scope to valorise and work productively with Indigenous relational ontologies, and holistic health. In this sense, health phenomena (illness experience, risk, determinants, interventions, etc.) and mental health conditions cannot be separated from the materiality of cultural and spiritual life (Dudgeon, Bray, D'Costa, & Walker, 2017). Aboriginal people view health through a cosmology that recognises interconnectedness in ways western health has failed to do so; 'their contexts for health issues are also diverse, requiring a more holistic and informed response to the ongoing effects of colonisation' (Sherwood & Edwards, 2006, p. 178). This is a move away from the dominant western approach that continues to manage Aboriginal health through a linear spectrum of illness and disease. Thinking posthumanism *with* the pluriverse concept enhances the utility of the theoretical and methodological tools in relation to the 'cultural interface' (Nakata, 2007) and the cultural and political imaginaries produced from in-between, borderland spaces (Anzaldúa & Keating, 2015).

The third strategy is to take up feminist, Indigenous and decolonial insights that we understand and experience the world from particular historical, cultural and social contexts, and account for how *ontological situatedness co-constitutes posthuman research* (Sundberg, 2014; Todd, 2016). This notion builds on the sociological tradition of researcher reflexivity and informs how health researchers orientate to 'more-than-human' research methodologies. In this special issue, Gibson et al. (2021) and Setchell et al. (2021) use iterative, exploratory, collaborative research processes. They identify how team members have a variety of social, cultural and disciplinary positions, and also take up a range of positions in their encounters with the health care system. Both papers endeavour to articulate and consider how their multiple positions shaped the research processes. This reflective effort led Gibson et al. (2021) to conclude 'there are inevitable gaps and interpretations that led us to map assemblages in ways that are always and necessarily partial' (p. 13). Acknowledging the specific, partial assemblages which emerge from research processes is a positive consequence of accounting for how researchers' situatedness co-composes posthuman research processes. In addition, we draw attention to the decolonial and Indigenous scholars who emphasise the importance of including explicit consideration of relatedness with colonial systems and western dominance. As Moreton-Robinson (2013) identifies, for western scholars, making self-location explicit necessarily involves considering their own relation to western dominance and the colonising system, and unpacking how colonial discourses have shaped a person's cultural identity and the roles and positions available to them. For Lawhon et al. (2016), this entailed years of collaboratively naming and exploring self-location via the strategy of unlearning: 'a partial, reflexive process of identifying the ways our conceptualisations of the world are unselfconsciously bounded and invisibly contingent' (Lawhon et al., 2016, p. 1614). Catherine Walsh explains how making oneself visible in the 'thinking with' is a vital component in creating a decolonial intention, 'in all aspects of my relational being-becoming' (Mignolo & Walsh, 2018, p. 21). For Kim, it has been necessary to interrogate how their position as a white, settler

Australian shaped the colonising gestures in their work with posthuman thinking. Writing the editorial propelled further questioning about the affordances of whiteness in academic knowledge production, and the ongoing need 'to exercise reflexivity on academic performativity, in terms of how space is taken up and granted' (Puwar, 2020, p. 552). For Simone, engaging with posthuman perspectives, Indigenous and decolonial scholars has contributed to a questioning of the privilege afforded to white settler knowledge, as well as a recognition of the incommensurability of different ontologies, sovereignty and identity connected to country (Moreton-Robinson, 2013).

Staying with the dilemma of the remade human

This editorial traces how it is productive for health sociology to stay with the dilemma of the remade human and to maintain a questioning orientation along the lines enacted by Seear and Lenton (2021) in this special issue, who ask, 'Does the challenge to humanism that we have described sometimes have costs? We want to hold open this possibility in the analysis that follows' (p. 3). We suggest staying with this tension by bringing close examination to bear on the political consequences of the 'problem' of the remade human in their contexts, *and* how posthuman conceptual and methodological tools co-create the remade human. The posthuman shift from the agentic, sovereign individual to the subject who emerges from socio-material practices furthers projects of political interest to health sociology. It enables health sociologists to avoid attributing blame and pathologising associated with individualised accounts of health and illbeing (McLeod, 2017), and take a distributed range of agencies into account when investigating and making interventions into health care provision, evaluation, intervention and policy-making. The shift in attention from the agentic individual, to the agentic capacities of assemblages, allows ethical examination in addition to inquiry supported by humanistic models of ethics which feature the intentional moral human subject (McLeod, 2014b). In addition, health processes and experience can be understood beyond the binaries of nature/culture; mind/body; cognitive/affective, thus challenging the dualisms of modernity and contributing to social and ecological justice. Although posthumanism enables health sociologists to progress particular agendas, we emphasise the value of further problematising the posthuman decentring of the human and bringing sustained attention to bear on the ethical and political implications of this approach to knowledge-making in health.

Extending posthuman perspectives on health leads us to consider the proximate ethical and political frameworks that co-create research assemblages. Drawing on decolonial, feminist and Indigenous scholarship, we suggest orientating to posthuman thought as a provincial (Meghji, 2021; Mignolo & Walsh, 2018), pluriversal (Blaser & de la Cadena, 2018; Mignolo, 2000), and situated (Moreton-Robinson, 2013; Todd, 2016) endeavour enables explicitly engaging with, and accounting for, the political and ethical frameworks which accompany posthuman thinking – particularly the Anglo-European political and ethical frameworks. This in turn, allows posthuman knowledge-making to participate more purposefully in philosophical debates about who counts as human and who does not.

These epistemic tensions are not easily resolved but they work to animate the conversations between post/de/colonial logics, Indigenous non-dualistic relational ontologies and posthuman health sociology. Such conversations are required if posthuman health sociology is to contribute in a productive way to the decolonising of Aboriginal health, which positions Aboriginal people as experts in, owners of, their health (Prehn & Ezzy, 2020). There are resonances here with pluriversal perspectives that Kwok (2020, p. 129) proposes, as they enable 'subaltern' standpoints to be heard. A provincial, pluriversal, situated posthuman thought facilitates the kind of shift Pang (2021) observes is necessary in relation to Chinese philosophical concepts about embodiment: 'to recognise Chinese knowers as intellectual subjects, and to acknowledge New Confucianism as a legitimate source of knowledge for moving beyond conventional approaches of understanding dualistic bodily practices' (pp. 8–9). This orientation has the potential to strengthen how posthuman health sociology deploys race as a critical category of analysis. In turn, contributing to the capacity of posthuman health sociology to participate in the crucial project of articulating the intersections between race, racism and health (Watego, Sing & Macoun 2021).

To conclude this introduction to the special issue we point to the possibilities of posthuman health sociology for providing an orientation to forms of political action produced through engagement with different voices, human and nonhuman bodies and advocacy for the marginalised perspectives of those affected. As Seear and Lenton (2021) have suggested, engaging with affected communities can mobilise research to shape better outcomes from movements between medicine and subjects. Pienaar et al. (2021) also point to the importance of designing public health approaches which are responsive to, and learn from, the care practices people from diverse publics are already undertaking. Bringing a pluriversal, provincial and situated perspective to posthuman thinking orients the framework to conversations with multiple epistemologies, as opposed to a universalised application of theory to all contexts.

Thank you to all the reviewers, editors and authors who made this special issue possible.

References

Alaimo, S. (2017). *Gender: matter*. Farmington Hills, Mich: MacMillan Press.

Anzaldúa, G., & Keating, A. (2015). *Light in the dark/luz en lo oscuro: Rewriting identity, spirituality, reality*. Durham and London: Duke University Press.

Arnold, C., Atchison, J., & McKnight, A. (2021). Reciprocal relationships with trees: Rekindling Indigenous wellbeing and identity through the Yuin ontology of oneness. *Australian Geographer, 52* (2), 131–147.

Barad, K. (2007). *Meeting the universe halfway: Quantum physics and the entanglement of matter and meaning*. Durham and London: Duke University Press.

Barad, K. (2012). Nature's queer performativity. *Kvinder, Køn & Forskning, 1–2*, 25–53. doi.org/10.7146/kkf.v0i1-2.28067

Barad, K. (2015). Transmaterialities: Trans*/matter/realities and queer political imaginings. GLQ: *A Journal of Lesbian and Gay Studies, 21*(2–3), 387–422.

Blaser, M., & de la Cadena, M. (2018). Pluriverse: Proposals for a world of many worlds. In M. de la Cadena & M. Blaser (Eds.), *A world of many worlds* (pp. 1–22). Durham and London: Duke University Press.

Braidotti, R. (2020). 'We' are in this together, but we are not one and the same. *Journal of Bioethical Inquiry, 17* (4), 465–469.

Coffey, J. (2020). Assembling wellbeing: Bodies, affects and the 'conditions of possibility' for wellbeing. *Journal of Youth Studies*. doi:10.1080/13676261.2020.1844171

Cozza, M., Bruzzone, S., & Crevani, L. (2021). Materialities of elderly care: Caring together/apart in the political economy of caring apparatus. *Health Sociology Review, 30*(3), 1–15. doi:10.1080/14461242.2021.1976067.

de La Bellacasa, M. P. (2017). *Matters of care: Speculative ethics in more than human worlds*. Minneapolis: University of Minnesota Press.

Dennis, F., & Farrugia, A. (2017). Materialising drugged pleasures: Practice, politics, care. *The International Journal on Drug Policy, 49*, 86–91. https://doi.org/10.1016/j.drugpo.2017.10.001

Dudgeon, P., Bray, A., D'Costa, B., & Walker, R. (2017). Decolonising psychology: Validating social and emotional wellbeing. *Australian Psychologist, 52*(4), 316–325. https://doi.org/10.1111/ap.12294

Duff, C. (2015). Governing drug use otherwise: For an ethics of care. *Journal of Sociology, 51*(1), 81–96.

Fox, N. J., & Alldred, P. (2016). Sociology, environment and health: A materialist approach. *Public Health, 141*, 287–293. doi:10.1016/j.puhe.2016.09.015.

Fullagar, S. (2017). Post-qualitative inquiry and the new materialist turn: Implications for sport, health and physical culture research. *Qualitative Research in Sport, Exercise and Health, 9*(2), 247–257. doi:10.1080/2159676X.2016.1273896

Fullagar, S., O'Brien, W., & Pavlidis, A. (2019). *Feminism and a vital politics of depression and recovery.* London: Palgrave MacMillan.

Gibson, B. E., Fadyl, J. K., Terry, G., Waterworth, K., Mosleh, D., & Kayes, N. M. (2021). A posthuman decentring of person-centred care. *Health Sociology Review, Advanced online publication.* doi:10.1080/14461242.2021.1975555

Hörl, E. (2017). Introduction to general ecology: The ecologization of thinking (N. F. Schott, Trans.). In E. Hörl & J. Burton (Eds.), *General ecology: The new ecological paradigm* (pp. 1–74). London: Bloomsbury Academic.

Joronen, M., & Häkli, J. (2017). Politicizing ontology. *Progress in Human Geography, 41*(5), 561–579. https://doi.org/10.1177/0309132516652953

Kwok, H. (2020). Beyond the anti-racist reason: A postcolonial perspective on pandemic politics. *Health Sociology Review, 29*(2), 122–130. doi:10.1080/14461242.2020.1785320

Lawhon, M., Silver, J., Ernstson, H., & Pierce, J. (2016). Unlearning [un]located ideas in the provincialization of urban theory. *Regional studies, 50*(9), 1611–1622. http://doi.org/10.1080/00343404.2016.1162288

López, A. J. (2018). Contesting the material turn; or, the persistence of agency. *The Cambridge Journal of Postcolonial Literary Inquiry, 5*(3), 371–386. doi.org/10.1017/pli.2018.14.

Lupton, D., & Willis, K. (2021). *The COVID-19 crisis: Social perspectives.* Routledge.

Matthewman, S., & Huppatz, K. (2020). A sociology of Covid-19. *Journal of Sociology, 56*(4), 675–683. doi.org/10.1177/1440783320939416

Mcallum, T., & Rose, J. (2021). Domestic violence, coercive control and mental health in a pandemic: Disenthralling the ecology of the domestic. *Health Sociology Review, 30*(3). *Advance online publication.*

McLeod, K. (2014a). Orientating to assembling: Qualitative inquiry for more- than-human-worlds. *International Journal of Qualitative Methods, 13,* 377–394. doi.org/10.1177/160940691401300120.

McLeod, K. (2014b). The missing work of collaboration: Using assemblages to rethink antidepressant action. *Contemporary Drug Problems, 41,* 109–142. doi.org/10.1177/009145091404100106.

McLeod, K. (2017). *Wellbeing machine: How health emerges from the assemblages of everyday life.* Durham: Carolina Academic Press. ISBN 978-1-61163-705-2.

McLeod, K., Moore, R., Robinson, D., Ozkul, D., Ciftci, S., & Vincent, K. (2020). Using the pluriverse concept to critique eurocentrism in education. *Journal of Applied Learning & Teaching, 3*(Special Issue No. 1), 30–39. doi.org/10.37074/jalt.2020.3.s1.4.

Meghji, A. (2021). *Decolonising sociology.* Cambridge, UK: Polity.

Mignolo, W. (2000). *Local histories/global designs: Coloniality, subaltern knowledges, and border thinking.* Princeton, New Jersey: Princeton University Press.

Mignolo, W. D. (2005). *The idea of Latin America.* Hoboken, New Jersey: Blackwell

Mignolo, W., & Walsh, C. (2018). *On decoloniality: Concepts, analytics, praxis.* Durham and London: Duke University Press.

Moreton-Robinson, A. (2013). Towards an Australian Indigenous women's standpoint theory. *Australian Feminist Studies, 28*(78), 331–347. doi.org/10.1080/08164649.2013.876664.

Nakata, M. (2007). The cultural interface. *The Australian Journal of Indigenous Education, 36,* 7–14. doi.org/10.1017/S1326011100004646.

Pang, B. (2021). The postmonolingual turn: Rethinking embodiment with new confucianism in bodily education and research. *Sport, Education and Society.* doi:10.1080/13573322.2021.1953461

Pape, M. (2021). Lost in translation? Beyond sex as a biological variable in animal research. *Health Sociology Review,* Advance online publication. doi:10.1080/14461242.2021.1969981

Paur, J. (2017). *Terrorist assemblages: Homonationalism in queer times.* Durham and London: Duke University Press.

Pienaar, K., Flore, J., Power, J., & Murphy, D. (2021). Making publics in a pandemic: Posthuman relationalities, 'viral' intimacies and COVID-19. *Health Sociology Review,* Advance online publication. doi:10.1080/14461242.2021.1961600

Prehn, J., & Ezzy, D. (2020). Decolonising the health and well-being of aboriginal men in Australia. *Journal of Sociology, 56*(2), 151–166. doi.org/10.1177/1440783319856618.

Puwar, N. (2020). Puzzlement of a deja vu: Illuminaries of the global South. *The Sociological Review, 68*(3), 540–556. doi.org/10.1177/0038026119890254.

Pyyhtinen, O. (2016). *More-than-human sociology: A new sociological imagination.* New York: Springer.

Rosiek, J., Snyder, J., & Pratt, S. (2020). The new materialisms and Indigenous theories of non-human agency: Making the case for respectful anti-colonial engagement. *Qualitative Inquiry, 26*(3–4), 331–346. doi:10.1177/1077800419830135

Schulz, K. A. (2017). Decolonizing political ecology: Ontology, technology and 'critical' enchantment. *Journal of Political Ecology, 24*(1), 125–143. doi:https://doi.org/10.2458/v24i1.20789

Seear, K., & Lenton, E. (2021). Becoming posthuman: Hepatitis C, the race to elimination and the politics of remaking the subject. *Health Sociology Review, Advance online publication*, doi:10.1080/14461242.2021.1971102

Setchell, J., Olson, R., Turpin, M., Costa, N., Barlott, T., O'Halloran, K., … Hodges, P. (2021). Afflexivity in post-qualitative inquiry: Prioritising affect and reflexivity in the evaluation of a health information website. *Health Sociology Review*, doi:10.1080/14461242.2021.1976068

Sherwood, J., & Edwards, T. (2006). Decolonisation: A critical step for improving Aboriginal health. *Contemporary Nurse, 22*(2), 178–190. doi:10.5172/conu.2006.22.2.178

Sundberg, J. (2014). Decolonizing posthumanist geographies. *Cultural Geographies, 2*(1), 33–47.

Todd, Z. (2016). An Indigenous feminist's take on the ontological turn: 'Ontology' is just another word for colonialism. *Journal of Historical Sociology, 29*, 4– 22. doi:10.1111/johs.12124

Tuhiwai Smith, L. (2012). *Decolonizing methodologies: Research and Indigenous peoples*. London: Zed Books.

Vitellone, N. (2017). *Social science of the syringe: A sociology of injecting drug use* (1st ed.). London: Routledge.

Watego, C., Singh, D., & Macoun, A. (2021). *Partnership for justice in health: Scoping paper on race, racism and the Australian health system, discussion paper*. Melbourne: The Lowitja Institute. doi:10.48455/sdrt-sb97.

Weheliye, S. (2014). *Habeas viscus: Racializing assemblages, biopolitics, and black feminist theories of the human*. Durham and London: Duke University Press.

Willcox, M., Hickey-Moody, A., & Harris, A. M. (2021). Isol-AID, art and wellbeing: Posthuman community amid COVID-19. In D. Lupton & K. Willis (Eds.), *The COVID-19 Crisis* (pp. 115–127). London: Routledge.

Wynter, S. (2003). Unsettling the coloniality of being/power/truth/freedom: Towards the Human, after man, its overrepresentation – An argument. *CR: The New Centennial Review, 3*(3), 257–337. doi:10.1353/ncr.2004.0015

Wynter, S., & McKittrick, K. (2015). Unparalleled catastrophe for our species? Or, to give humanness a different future: Conversations. In K. McKittrick (Ed.), *Sylvia Wynter: On being human as praxis* (pp. 9–89). Durham and London: Duke University Press.

Zembylas, M. (2018). The entanglement of decolonial and posthuman perspectives: Tensions and implications for curriculum and pedagogy in higher education. *Parallax, 24*(3), 254–267. doi:10.1080/13534645.2018.1496577

Becoming posthuman: hepatitis C, the race to elimination and the politics of remaking the subject

Kate Seear and Emily Lenton

ABSTRACT

Hepatitis C has long been a public health problem in Australia. 'Revolutionary' new drugs with the potential to cure hepatitis C have now emerged. The Australian government has invested heavily in them, and has an ambitious goal to eliminate hepatitis C by 2030. Numerous shifts in policy and practice are required if the elimination agenda is to be realised. This paper explores the significance of these shifts. We ask: what is the race to elimination *doing with the subject*? We argue that the race to elimination can be understood, simultaneously, as a *product* of posthuman forces, capable of being analysed using the theoretical tools made available via the posthuman turn; producing an *intervention* in what it means to be human; and generating a *dilemma* for people who use (or used) drugs, people with hepatitis C, and posthuman scholarship. In drawing out these issues, we aim to: trace the significant developments underway in hepatitis C medicine and raise awareness of them; encourage reflection on the consequences of these developments; and invite reflections on what might be lost when the human is remade by hepatitis C medicine.

Introduction

Hepatitis C is a blood-borne virus (BBV). Transmission largely occurs in the context of injecting drug use, through the sharing of needles and syringes or ancillary injecting equipment (Fraser & Seear, 2011). For many years, the most widely available form of treatment for hepatitis C was known as 'combination therapy'. Under this regime, only about 3000 people annually commenced treatment in Australia (Hellard, 2014). Drugs were taken for 24–48 weeks, with the length of treatment dependent on a range of factors including viral genotype (Hopwood & Treloar, 2007). Combination therapy was notoriously onerous because of the wide range of reported side effects (Fraser & Seear, 2011), and many people discontinued treatment before completion of the regime (Hopwood & Treloar, 2007). A new generation of hepatitis C treatment known as direct-acting antivirals, or DAAs, then emerged. The reported benefits of DAAs are numerous and include a treatment period reduced from 24–28 weeks to 8–12 weeks, and dramatic improvements in cure rates – from 40% for combination therapy to over 95% (European Association for the Study of the Liver, 2020). Fewer serious side effects are reported (Asselah, Boyer, Saadoun, Martinot-Peignoux, & Marcellin, 2016), and treatment is more tolerable. DAAs were almost immediately lauded as 'revolutionary' (e.g. Gane, 2014; Martinello, Hajarizadeh, & Dore, 2018). They bring the possibility of large numbers of those affected being cured, or the possibility of viral elimination altogether.

The World Health Organization has announced an ambitious goal to eliminate hepatitis C by 2030, and Australia is one of the only countries to have adopted it (Commonwealth Department of Health, 2018; World Health Organization, 2016). In 2015, Australia offered universal access to DAAs, listing them on the Pharmaceutical Benefits Scheme, making it a world leader in treatment (Dore, 2017). There is considerable global interest in whether Australia can eliminate hepatitis C. Accessing, screening, diagnosing and treating people is key to this ambitious project, and numerous shifts in policy and practice are required to realise the elimination agenda. The 'race to elimination' has indeed driven dramatic changes in the national policy landscape, including new models of care and micro-elimination strategies (Lazarus et al., 2018). There are also shifts in models of testing and treatment, and in the way that individual rights are viewed, including the fundamental right not to undergo any medical procedure without one's full and fully informed consent (Berg, Appelbaum, Lidz, & Parker, 2001). This paper explores the significance of these shifts. We ask: what is the race to elimination *doing with the subjects of hepatitis C medicine*, many of whom are people who inject (or have previously injected) drugs? And how might we assess these developments?

In this paper, we argue that multiple, entangled, mutually reinforcing shifts in testing, treatment and approaches to patient rights are underway, and that these processes raise urgent ethical and political questions for healthcare in Australia. We argue that the race to elimination can be understood, simultaneously, as a *product* of posthuman forces, capable of being analysed using the theoretical tools made available via the posthuman turn; producing an *intervention* in what it means to be human, and generating a *dilemma* for people who use (or used) drugs, people with hepatitis C, and for a posthuman scholarship. This dilemma has some parallels with one identified by David Moore and Suzanne Fraser (2006) in their previous work on subject positions in harm reduction, but differs in important ways, as we will explain. Overall, we argue that the remaking of the subject that is taking place in Australian healthcare introduces costs (such as invasions of bodily integrity, autonomy, and privacy), which can be hugely troubling for people who use drugs and people with hepatitis C. In drawing out these processes and dilemmas, we aim to do three things. First, to trace the significant developments underway in hepatitis C medicine, so as to raise awareness of them. Second, to encourage policy-makers, practitioners, researchers and others to think carefully about the consequences that might follow these developments, especially (but not only) for people who use/have used drugs. Third, we invite reflections on what might be lost when the human is remade by hepatitis C medicine, and consider possible broader implications of this.

Background

Most countries around the world have legal regimes that criminalise the use, possession and supply of certain substances. A key logic underpinning prohibition is the notion that drugs produce various predictable effects and harms (Fraser & Moore, 2011b). These harms include hepatitis C, with the virus sometimes described as an inevitable and predictable effect of drug use (Rhodes & Treloar, 2008), even though its association is complex and far from certain (Fraser & Seear, 2011). This idea – of drug effects as consistent and predictable – is frequently mobilised in defence of drug prohibition. It is also contested and controversial, and has been the subject of much critical alcohol and other drug (AOD) scholarship. Critical AOD scholarship mobilises poststructuralist, feminist, queer, new-materialist and more-than-human or posthuman philosophies. Collectively, such work challenges the claim that drug effects are singular, predictable, stable and fixed (i.e. that drug use is always already harmful), emphasising instead the multiplicity, unpredictability, instability and inconsistency of drug effects (Fraser & Moore, 2011b). This work argues that drug effects, harms and other realities are not *inherent* to substances. It seeks to shift the 'unit of analysis' (Duff, 2017) from drugs 'themselves' to 'drug events' (e.g. Dennis, 2019; Farrugia 2017; Malins 2017; Dilkes-Frayne and Duff 2017; Fitzgerald 2015) and 'assemblages' (Deleuze & Parnet, 1987) of material, human and non-human forces in their 'intra-actions' (Barad, 2007; Fraser 2006). Such work invites us to think about harms associated with drugs as posthuman: always already the product of multiple mutually constitutive forces operating in intra-action, and to think about subjects, objects and agency differently; not as vested only or purely in humans, but in a 'range of different kinds of actors' (Cohn & Lynch, 2017, p. 286).

These approaches allow us to conceptualise harm 'as a property of the assemblage and not of any one discrete body therein [e.g. the drug or the person who uses drugs]' (Duff, 2014, p. 634). Such 'assemblage thinking' (Deleuze & Parnet, 1987) disrupts dominant ideas about drugs and those who use them, and challenges prevailing approaches to agency, responsibility and causality. It also decentres the human. In this sense, posthuman approaches open up an important political space, pushing back against the foundational logics of drug law, policy and related fields of practice. Posthuman theories can also be mobilised when analysing hepatitis C acquired through other means, such as blood transfusions, although relevant political issues will differ. In this paper, we want to reflect on what becomes of the subject, once we start to think through phenomena using posthuman theory. Does the challenge to humanism that we have described above sometimes have costs? We want to hold open this possibility in the analysis that follows, through a detailed exploration of the rapidly evolving contours of hepatitis C medicine. Before we come to this analysis, however, we want to introduce one further set of ideas that are relevant to the analysis we will undertake in this paper.

Theory and method

The question of the subject is always pertinent but it is especially so in AOD scholarship and scholarship that pertains to harm reduction. One of the most comprehensive analyses of the 'drug-using subject' is David Moore and Suzanne Fraser's (2006) work on the subject of harm reduction. Although harm reduction policy and practice has done much to improve the lives of people who use drugs, by, for instance, preventing transmission of blood-borne viruses such as hepatitis C, and helping to prevent drug overdose deaths, harm reduction may still be flawed in some ways. Taking this as their starting point, Moore and Fraser (2006) argue that harm reduction inscribes a neoliberal subject, positioning people who use drugs as autonomous, rational, independent and calculating. One problem with this inscription is that it fails to account for the many ways that agency is constrained. As they explain,

> this failure risks diverting policy and practice away from structural issues and the resulting unequal distribution of resources, limiting our conception of effective strategies for harm reduction. (2006, p. 3036)

Inscriptions of the subject as autonomous, rational, independent and calculating can responsibilise people for harms associated with drugs, such as the transmission of hepatitis C through the sharing of needles, while structural failings, such as the lack of sterile needles and syringes for people who need them, can be overlooked. The subject is put at the centre of drug harms in this way, and risks being positioned as a 'failure' (Fraser & Seear, 2011). The neoliberal subject also had benefits, however. Constituting subjects as autonomous, rational, independent and calculating might be empowering for some people who use drugs, given that this subject position carries benefits such as trust and legitimation. This, they argue, constitutes 'a dilemma' for harm reduction policy and practice. How should we react when faced with this simultaneously beneficial and harmful move?

To answer this question, Moore and Fraser turn to Judith Butler's (2004:, p. 227) work on how feminists might respond to the (white, male, heteronormative) subject of liberalism. As Butler explains, to

> question the foundationalism of that category [of the subject] is not the same thing as doing away with it all together. Moreover, it is not to deny its usefulness, or even its necessity. To question the subject is to put at risk what we know, and to do it not for the thrill of the risk, but because we have already been put into question as subjects. We have already, as women, been severely doubted: do our words carry meaning? Are we capable of consent? Is our reasoning functioning like that of men? Are we part of the universal community of human kind?

Moore and Fraser (2006) argue that this approach – of putting at risk what we know – has value for harm reduction. It is possible, as Butler suggests, to be both skeptical towards the liberal subject and to acknowledge its strategic value. This leads Moore and Fraser to conclude that:

> we must reject any dream of discovering a 'pure' location from which to construct the 'ideal' subject of harm reduction. There is no such place. Our intention in this paper has not been to identify and recommend such a location but to spell out the processes of subjectification at work in harm reduction, and the implications of the forms of subject produced. In doing so, we hope to prompt insights into future directions for the subject of harm reduction. (Moore & Fraser, 2006, p. 3045)

Moore and Fraser's focus was on the specific question of what harm reduction was doing to the subject, and what costs and benefits flowed from the predominantly neoliberal subject of harm reduction. Their work took place before the emergence of the race to elimination, where new subject positions and political questions are emerging. It is vital that we trace these and consider their implications. Indeed, we know from previous work on hepatitis C (Fraser & Seear, 2011) that any shifts in hepatitis C medicine, including treatment policy and practice, shape shifts in subject formulations, given the co-constitutive relationship between medicine and subjects (see also Lancaster & Rhodes, in press). This paper takes up these issues and asks: what is the race to elimination *doing with the subject*? And how might we assess these developments? In what follows, we trace a series of important shifts happening in the landscape of hepatitis C policy and practice. In order to undertake this analysis, we collected and analysed the national policy and strategy documents on hepatitis C since the first national strategy was introduced 20 years ago. Paying careful attention to key phrases and words used throughout these texts, we assessed how the virus and treatment were described over time, how strategies and policy priorities evolved, and how people with hepatitis C were described alongside these shifts. We then searched for recent research on novel strategies and practices designed to further the elimination agenda, exploring how the subject and their rights were described. Our familiarity with work of this kind was also informed by our many years working within the field of hepatitis C. We argue that the race to elimination can be understood as: a *product* of posthuman forces, capable of being analysed using the theoretical tools made available via the posthuman turn; producing an *intervention* in what it means to be human; and generating a *dilemma* for subjects similar to the one surfaced by Moore and Fraser in their critique of harm reduction. This dilemma is important to the posthuman turn in drug scholarship, and to posthuman health scholarship more broadly.

The shifting landscape of hepatitis C

Shifting treatments

As noted earlier, the treatment landscape has shifted dramatically in Australia over the last few years, with the advent of DAAs. Initial take-up of DAA treatments was strong, but has declined over time (MacLachlan, Smith, Towell, & Cowie, 2020). This plateauing in treatment uptake has meant that Australia's commitment to eliminating hepatitis C by 2030 looks increasingly less easy to honour. There are numerous possible reasons for this, including that hepatitis C can be asymptomatic, and that there can be challenges in connecting with affected and undiagnosed populations (Martinello & Matthews, 2015). People who inject drugs are a highly stigmatised and often marginalised population (e.g. Fraser et al., 2017; Lancaster, Seear, & Ritter, 2018; Lloyd, 2010), and do not always trust health care systems, including digital systems (Newman et al., 2020; Treloar, Rance, & Backmund, 2013). Thus, the availability of DAAs will not, in itself, be enough to cure everyone, and more 'innovative' methods are needed (Wright et al., 2019). These innovations have manifested in numerous ways. For example, hepatitis C testing used to have an 'exceptional' status in which detailed pre-test counselling was required. This requirement has now been removed, as testing has sought to be normalised (Johnson & Lenton, 2017). These forces have added pressure to other areas of policy and practice, provoking other shifts designed to support Australia's elimination agenda, including changes in strategy.

Shifting strategies

Australia's approach to hepatitis C has been governed, since 1999, by a series of national strategies, complemented by policies including the *National Drug Strategy 2017–2026* (Commonwealth Department of Health, 2017) and state and territory strategies. The first *National Hepatitis C Strategy 1999–2000 to 2003–2004* had two primary aims, which were 'to reduce the transmission of hepatitis C in Australia' and 'to minimise the personal and social impacts of hepatitis C infection' (Commonwealth Department of Health and Aged Care, 2000, p. 1). An important conceptual move occurred in the second *National Hepatitis C Strategy 2005–2008*. Although the strategy retained a focus on individuals and individual responsibility, it also emphasised the possibility that treatment of individuals could have benefits for the population as a whole. To this end, the strategy noted that cure 'not only improves quality of life for those who successfully undergo treatment, but also reduces the risk of passing the virus on to others' (Commonwealth of Australia, 2005, p. 17). Later, calls emerged for treatment rates to be trebled (Treloar & Rhodes, 2009). These moves were consolidated in later strategies, through calls for a stronger public health response to the virus (WHO, 2016) and via the adoption of a 'treatment as prevention' approach (known as TasP). First used within the context of HIV, treatment as prevention sees 'treatment as a tool for limiting spread of an infection in generalised epidemics in a particular setting' (Hajarizadeh et al., 2016, p. 317). The idea is that testing and treatment have benefits for individuals, who will be diagnosed, treated and cured, and populations, as cure helps prevent 'onward transmission' (Hellard et al., 2014). TasP now figures explicitly in the national strategy (Commonwealth Department of Health, 2018), with new treatments described as having 'the potential to reduce overall hepatitis C incidence as the population of people living with hepatitis C diminishes' (Commonwealth Department of Health, 2018, p. 23). The World Health Organization (2017) has also acknowledged the value of TasP. The current national strategy also embraces elimination of hepatitis C as a key goal (Commonwealth Department of Health, 2018). Testing and treatment are priority areas, and the WHO (2016) established time bound targets for testing, adding further systemic pressures.

These shifts instantiate the primacy of the individual subject, by prioritising locating, testing and treating *individuals*, and the possibility of *individual transformation through cure*. This apparent valorisation of the individual appears elsewhere in the national strategy, as where a commitment to the human rights of people with hepatitis C, 'including the right to the confidential and sensitive handling of personal and medical information' is now included (Commonwealth Department of Health, 2018). We argue that the picture is more complicated, however. A decade ago, Fraser and Moore (2011a:, p. 377) wrote critically of the rush to increase treatment rates, describing a 'growing sense that treatment comprises an important part of the response to the scale of the epidemic'. They argued that although treatment was onerous and harmful for many people, potentially not suited to their individual needs and circumstances, it was nevertheless thought to be 'warranted as part of a strategy for helping to reduce overall transmission, and therefore prevalence, rates' (2011a, p. 377). They described this move as homogenising, arguing that such responses:

> risk treating affected people as epidemiological units bereft of individual differences and circumstances, and their personal interests as indistinguishable from those of society as a whole, despite their evident exclusion from many of the rewards offered by society. (2011a, p. 377)

Of course, Fraser and Moore's critique pre-dated the emergence of DAAs. This renders some aspects of their analysis less relevant for DAAs, given that they are more successful and tolerable. The notion, however, that the medicalisation of hepatitis C was conflating individual interests with public health outcomes was an important concern, becoming only more important with the passage of time and the race to elimination. Acknowledging that cure can be profoundly beneficial for many people, others note that public health outcomes and priorities do not necessarily matter to publics (Harris, Albers, & Swan, 2015). Moreover, both the TasP approach and some public health rhetoric can be stigmatising, alienating and unintentionally dehumanising, especially where individuals are constituted as 'transmitters'. Through all of this, the 'individual – their needs, fears and desires – slips from focus' (Harris et al., 2015, p. 965).

This trend has arguably gathered pace in the years since, with significant investment in elimination, and shifting strategies and practices. Somewhat paradoxically, the advent of DAAs and the elimination agenda is generating a shift *away from* the individual. Starting at least with the second *National Strategy's* aforementioned homogenising move as identified by Fraser and Moore (2011a), the subject of hepatitis C medicine is being remade. This remaking is a product of the elimination 'assemblage', which includes drugs, epidemiological measures and methods, policy documents, government resources, pharmaceutical companies, refrigerators to store drugs, public health targets, models and strategies, trucks, scientists, nurses and doctors, laboratories, devices, needles, outreach vans, hospitals and doctors' waiting rooms, as well as the effects produced by the imagined elimination 'boundary' of the nation state (Seear, Fraser, Farrugia, & Valentine, in press) entangled in intra-action (Barad, 2007). Through these intra-actions, individuals are conflated with publics, personal interests become national ones, and individuals are made relationally (i.e. where cure is important for subjects via connections to others, and the potential to reduce onward transmission). These changes bear some similarities to those underway in HIV medicine, including important changes in the 'nature' and 'criterion' of citizenship accompanying the pharmaceuticalisation of public health, and its potential to demarginalise and marginalise people living with HIV (Persson, Newman, Mao, & de Wit, 2016). Against all of this, certain obstacles – in the form of individual legal rights and medico-legal obligations – appear to stand in the way of the subject 'slipping' away (Harris et al., 2015) altogether. As we will see in the next section, even these vestiges of liberal humanism are giving way, raising urgent questions about the politics and ethics of the posthuman turn being wrought by hepatitis C medicine.

Shifting approaches to consent and rights

Testing and diagnosis are central to an imagined post-hepatitis C future. This requires people to first provide informed consent: typically defined as being met when a person develops a full appreciation of the benefits and risks of a proposed course of action, such as medical tests or treatment, and agrees to proceed (Berg et al., 2001). Informed consent is a legal requirement in Australia, enshrined in both the common law and statute (e.g. *Rogers v Whitaker* (1992) 175 CLR 479). It is therefore, an important precursor to diagnosis, treatment and cure, and a potential barrier to broader elimination efforts. As a transaction between putatively 'free and equal' persons, it is closely tied to individualism and humanism. The requirement that people provide informed consent prior to testing is acknowledged in the current national hepatitis C strategy, where it is stated that:

> The principles of quality testing in Australia include that *informed consent is required at all times*, including in custodial settings; and that testing is voluntary, accessible, non discriminatory, confidential and of clear benefit to the individual being tested. (Commonwealth Department of Health, 2018, p. 24; emphasis added)

Relevantly, the current national testing policy states that testing should be voluntary (Commonwealth of Australia, 2020). Later the policy says that: 'Informed consent for testing means that the person being tested agrees to be tested on the basis of understanding the testing procedures and the reasons for testing, and is able to assess the personal implications' (Commonwealth of Australia, 2020, p. 16). The WHO's best practice guidelines also note that 'informed consent should be tailored to an individual's gender, culture, health literacy and intellectual level' (2017, p. 7). This appears to instantiate the primacy of the individual subject, emphasising individual rights, bodily integrity and autonomy, the need to tailor explanations to individuals based on unique personal characteristics, and so on. The requirement for informed consent thus appears at odds with the more-than-human, homogenising and relational forces we described previously. However, both the rhetoric and operationalisation of consent are changing.

In Spain, for example, Andaluz et al. (2020) have argued that:

> In order to achieve [the elimination] objective, we must go beyond the routine treatment provided at our clinics and design new strategies for identifying infected patients, many of whom are unaware of their illness.

They position barriers to testing and treatment (including legal rights protections) as potentially unethical, arguing that 'not acting in the knowledge that an effective treatment is available could be considered as a failure to provide assistance' (Andaluz et al., 2020). Similar rhetoric can be found in Australia. For instance, some have noted that 'Australia is unlikely to meet the WHO targets unless the identification and testing of people exposed to hepatitis C are increased by 50%' (Scott et al., 2020). They go on to list a range of other methods for improving testing rates, including, for instance, 'introducing mandatory reporting of hepatitis C testing as key performance indicators for opioid substitution therapy clinics and prisons' (Scott et al., 2020, p. 369). These shifts in rhetoric, which are about how systems can be reformed and efforts to test scaled up, are complemented by important shifts in practice. These include novel strategies to locate people who have been lost to follow-up, including by waiving the requirement that they consent to being contacted after several years (Kracht et al., 2019) and other attempts to explore 'limited patient consent procedures' that make gaining consent for testing less onerous, potentially at the expense of patient autonomy (e.g. Crane, Henderson, & Chadwick, 2017). We are also seeing a shift from 'opt in' approaches, which require clear and affirmative action (e.g. verbally) to indicate consent, to 'opt out' approaches, which assume that a person consents unless they affirmatively indicate otherwise. Actively finding people by following up notification data, contract tracing and searching health records are some of the more recent strategies implemented to reach elimination targets (Stoové et al., 2020). This is happening in England, Ireland (Francis-Graham et al., 2019; O'Kelly, Byrne, Naughten, Bergin, & Williams, 2016), and Australia, including through the recent SEARCH study (Prince et al., 2021) in New South Wales. That study involved a novel method for locating, testing and treating Aboriginal and Torres Strait Islanders and overseas-born residents who might have hepatitis C. A team of researchers tested the previously stored blood samples of patients who had attended an emergency department for another medical reason (i.e. non-hepatitis C). They used an opt out method, through which posters and brochures in some 'common languages' (Prince et al., 2021) were placed around the emergency department, advising that people's stored blood might be retrospectively tested for hepatitis C. Around 5000 samples were tested in this way. This method was described as having 'removed barriers to testing' (Prince et al., 2021, p. 127).

Together, these practices have at least four important features. First, they involve less, and less direct, engagement with patients than in the past, manifesting a dilution in the substance of informed consent and its symbolic and literal value. There is a move away from detailed pre- and post-test counselling, changing the way the individual facing a test and/or diagnosis is treated, and reducing opportunities for care. Second, they utilise language and concepts that enact individuals and their rights as an impediment to testing and treatment. Although such moves are often said to be about advancing patient health and human rights (e.g. Prince et al., 2021), these moves are also tied to the elimination agenda. Although we acknowledge that comprehensive pre- and post-test conversations take time, is this reason in itself to take blood from someone, when/if they are unable to assess the possible benefits or risks of a positive diagnosis? Is the subject being made as less valuable, or differently, through such processes? Thirdly, individuals and their rights come to be constituted as problems for testing, cure and elimination. This has the potential to obscure other forces that might have influenced a decline in rates of testing and treatment, and to why people are 'lost to follow up'. These include persistent stigma and discrimination of people who use drugs in healthcare settings (Lancaster et al., 2018), a lack of trust in health care systems (Newman et al., 2020; Treloar et al., 2013), and a failure of treatment to live up to expectations (Madden, Hopwood, Neale, & Treloar, 2018a, 2018b; Whiteley, Whittaker, Elliott, & Cunningham-Burley, 2018). To date, debates about these developments tend to focus largely on narrowly bioethical questions, such as whether the benefits of testing and treatment outweigh the disadvantages and risks (e.g. Van Dijk, van Agt, & Drenth, 2020), including the risk of shock that one's blood has been tested without express permission, or the sense that one's privacy has been breached. We see these moves differently, however. They represent an erasure of humanist ideals and values, such as individual freedom, autonomy and integrity, and an intensification of the process by which the subject of hepatitis C medicine disappears from view, or becomes posthuman. To the extent that being conferred with such rights is understood to signal one's status as a valid, valued subject (i.e. as 'human'), the remaking of this right, and its apparent diminution, remakes the human.

Discussion: becoming posthuman

Across several iterations of national hepatitis C strategies, testing policies, other human and non-human forces including curative drugs, and processes pertaining to consent and rights, we are witnessing a set of vital shifts for people who live with hepatitis C/people who use drugs. These shifts are not simply about the availability of medicine, but shifts in how subjects are constituted, in relation to each other, drugs, medicine, medical policy, and the State. All of this is possible because medicine and subjects are co-constituting

(Fraser & Seear, 2011). Many of the shifts taking place in hepatitis C medicine appear subtle, as with shifts happening in relation to the specific way that 'opt in' approaches to consent have given way to 'opt out' approaches, or with the specifics of how opt out consent is being implemented (e.g. a conversation about testing, versus a flyer handed to a person, versus a poster hung on a wall). When these moves are analysed together, we see *a shift in how the subject of hepatitis C medicine is both perceived and enacted via the race to elimination.* As Fraser and Moore (2011a:, p. 377) observed nearly a decade ago, regarding the push to treat people who use drugs in order to prevent onward transmission, subjects appear as 'bereft of individual differences and circumstances' with 'their personal interests [...] indistinguishable from those of society as a whole'. We see something similar going on here. However, these developments have intensified significantly in the decade since Fraser and Moore (2011a) offered their critique, as elimination became entrenched through practice and policy. These logics have benefits and costs. Our point in this article is not to deny the benefits that flow from testing, treatment and cure, but to instead invite critical reflection on the rapidly changing version of subjecthood being made possible by DAAs and to encourage reflection regarding the various forces that are limiting ways of being and becoming with hepatitis C. A remaking that is simultaneously homogenising, humanising and dehumanising is underway, and we must attend to what this means for those affected.

Here, we want to reflect on what such tensions and movements *do with the human.* Can the subject who uses or who has ever used drugs be (or remain) 'human' in the face of a set of forces that position them and their interests as mere obstacles to other goals? What is the place of the subject in the midst of this web of forces? How does one live in a world dominated by a powerful national/global agenda? The specific changes we have traced in this paper can be seen as simultaneously: a *product* of more-than-human forces, an *intervention* in what it means to be human, and generative of a *dilemma* for people who use drugs, as well as for critical drug scholarship and posthuman scholarship more broadly. This dilemma has some parallels with that identified by Moore and Fraser (2006) in their previous work on the neoliberal subject of harm reduction, insofar as the subject positions inscribed in (or made available through) the elimination agenda have costs and benefits for people who use drugs. Here, the dilemma we identify is of a slightly different kind. The choice is not between the possibilities and limitations of neoliberal subjecthood but between humanism, which can create significant problems for people who fail to live up its normalising ideals, and posthumanism, which can erase the subject and much-needed protections. This generates new dilemmas for posthumanism in critical AOD and health scholarship. As we explained earlier, moves away from humanism are seen to have great analytic, symbolic and material power in AOD scholarship, positioning drug effects and forms of harm not as the product of individual subjects but of assemblages. But posthuman phenomena may not generate consistently valuable outcomes across different areas of policy and practice. The remaking of subjects in legal spheres can generate benefits that differ markedly from their remaking within medical ones. In the present setting, the remaking of the subject has a set of political effects that differ markedly from the effects that might flow in, say, research into the assemblage of the drug overdose event. On the one hand, the subject is remade in its relations to others, constituted as part of a national (or possibly global) collective, where bodies, affects and interests are entangled. The recognition that all people who use drugs are connected through the elimination effort together might be empowering, inspiring and galvanising, offering a sense of optimism and purpose via a relational, monistic worldview. This new way of understanding oneself and one's place in the world through medicine has the potential to confer new benefits, especially if it allows people who use drugs to move beyond the narrow confines of 'addicted' subjecthood. Under this approach, dependence gives way to interdependence, rather than independence, which was the subject position made available under neoliberalism (Moore & Fraser, 2006). But there are also problems with a version of subjecthood in which subjects are principally constituted via their relations to others and to broader public health goals. Whereas the value of posthumanism in AOD scholarship is its remaking of the subject as less responsible for forms of harm traditionally assigned to them as individuals, in the present context we see an erasure of rights and forms of care which are unquestionably precious to marginalised members of society, including people who use drugs and people with hepatitis C.

Conclusion

The remaking of the subject under elimination introduces costs (such as invasions of bodily integrity, autonomy, and privacy), which can be hugely troubling for people who use drugs and people with hepatitis C. These moves may also erode trust in medicine and undermine the elimination agenda, even as they advance it. The various risks and costs of such moves include: deterring people from treatment, if they feel their trust has been breached, or if they feel dehumanised in some way; the risk of re-infection, greater marginalisation and stigma, if people disengage with service providers; and the myriad of social, community and economic costs that may follow. As with the neoliberal subjects of Moore and Fraser's (2006) earlier work, we can find no simple answer to this dilemma. There is no 'pure location' from which to construct the ideal subject after the posthuman turn. There is a need, instead, to be attentive to what is happening under elimination, to ask whether all of these moves are essential, and to reflect on what they do. This problem is likely to intensify as Australia moves closer to its 2030 elimination deadline, encounters stepped targets for testing and treatment, and is subject to the watchful gaze of other nation States. All of this raises important and urgent questions about the place of individual interests, rights and ways of being in the face of cure, and a powerful national apparatus that is determined to eliminate the virus. It also has other implications for people with hepatitis C, affording 'revised notions of citizenship and social inclusion among people who inject drugs and others affected' by the virus (Rance, Rhodes, & Lancaster, 2021). We need to think with care about the gains and losses generated through the elimination agenda.

To conclude, we offer some speculative pathways for addressing some of the questions and challenges we have identified in this paper. First, we argue that meaningful engagement of affected communities is essential at all points of the policy development and implementation process. In policymaking and strategic planning, including in the push to upscale testing and treatment, more careful attention must be paid to the needs and rights of people with hepatitis C. It is important to think beyond the 2030 elimination goal, and to consider the risks that are introduced by subtle shifts in language, models of testing and treatment and changes to consent. These effects may be severe and long lasting for an already marginalised group. Ethics committees who are tasked with approving 'novel' or 'innovative' strategies for upscaling testing and treatment should be encouraged to consider the effects of remaking consent, beyond narrowly bioethical considerations of the kind we noted earlier. There is also value in considering a charter for better safeguarding patient rights in this context, including for the use and re-use of health records (Dencik, 2020), and to explore other measures that would protect the rights and interests of individuals concerning testing, diagnosis and treatment. Finally, researchers might seek to deliberately intervene in these dynamics (following Fraser, in press) and instigate change (Seear et al., in press) by conducting research expressly focussed on the needs, perspectives, experiences and rights of those affected by the elimination agenda. Such work allows us to attend more carefully to what is happening, and to shape movements between subjects and medicine to 'enact better outcomes' (Fraser, in press) for some of the most marginalised members of our community.

Disclosure statement

No potential conflict of interest was reported by the author(s).

Funding

The research reported in this paper is funded by the Australian Research Council (DP200100941).

ORCID

Kate Seear http://orcid.org/0000-0002-0886-7069

References

Andaluz, I., del Mar Arcos, M., Montero, M. D., Castillo, P., Martin-Carbonero, L., Garcia-Samaniego, J., & Olveira, A. (2020). Patients with hepatitis C lost to follow-up: Ethical-legal aspects and search results. *Revista Espanola de Enfermadades Digestivas (REED)*, *112*(7), 532–538.

Asselah, T., Boyer, N., Saadoun, D., Martinot-Peignoux, M., & Marcellin, P. (2016). Direct-acting antivirals for the treatment of hepatitis C virus infection: Optimizing current IFN-free treatment and future perspectives. *Liver International*, *36*, 47–57.

Barad, K. (2007). *Meeting the universe halfway: Quantum physics and the entanglement of matter and meaning*. Durham: Duke University Press.

Berg, J., Appelbaum, P., Lidz, C., & Parker, S. (2001). *Informed consent: Legal theory and clinical practice*. New Jersey: Oxford University Press.

Butler, J. (2004). *Undoing gender*. New York and London: Routledge.

Cohn, S., & Lynch, R. (2017). Posthuman perspectives: Relevance for a global public health. *Critical Public Health*, *27*(3), 285–292.

Commonwealth Department of Health. (2017). *National drug strategy 2017-2026*. Canberra: Commonwealth of Australia.

Commonwealth Department of Health. (2018). *Fifth national hepatitis C strategy 2018-2022*. Canberra: Department of Health.

Commonwealth Department of Health and Aged Care. (2000). *National hepatitis c strategy 1999-2000 to 2003-2004*. Canberra: Commonwealth Department of Health and Aged Care.

Commonwealth Department of Health and Ageing. (2005). *National hepatitis C strategy 2005-2008*. Canberra: Commonwealth of Australia.

Commonwealth of Australia. (2020). *National hepatitis c testing strategy.* Canberra: Commonwealth of Australia.

Crane, D., Henderson, E. J., & Chadwick, D. R. (2017). Exploring the acceptability of a 'limited patient consent procedure' for a proposed blood-borne virus screening programme: A Delphi consensus building technique. *BMJ Open, 7*(5), e015373.

Deleuze, G., & Parnet, C. (1987). *Dialogues.* London: Athlone Press.

Dencik, L. (2020). Advancing data justice in public health and beyond. *The American Journal of Bioethics, 20*(10), 32–33. doi:10.1080/15265161.2020.1806945

Dennis, F. (2019). *Injecting bodies in more-than-human worlds.* London: Routledge.

Dilkes-Frayne, E., & Duff, C. (2017). Tendencies and trajectories: The production of subjectivity in an event of drug consumption. *Environment and Planning D: Society and Space, 35*(5), 951–967.

Dore, G. (2017). Australia leads the world in hepatitis C treatment – What's behind its success? *The Conversation*, July 21.

Duff, C. (2014). The place and time of drugs. *International Journal of Drug Policy, 25*, 633–639.

Duff, C. (2017). Critical drug studies after the ontological turn. *Contemporary Drug Problems conference*, August, Helsinki: Finland.

European Association for the Study of the Liver. (2018). EASL recommendations on treatment of hepatitis C 2018. *Journal of Hepatology, 69*, 461–511.

Farrugia, A. (2017). Gender, reputation and regret: The ontological politics of Australian drug education. *Gender and Education, 29*(3), 281–298.

Fitzgerald, J. (2015). *Framing drug use: Bodies, space, economy and crime.* Basingstoke: Palgrave Macmillan.

Francis-Graham, S., Ekeke, N. A., Nelson, C. A., Lee, T. Y., El Haj, S., Rhodes, T., & Rosenberg, W. (2019). Understanding how, why, for whom, and under what circumstances opt-out blood-borne virus testing programmes work to increase test engagement and uptake within prison: A rapid-realist review. *BMC Health Services Research, 19*(1), 1–18.

Fraser, S. (2006). The chronotope of the queue: Methadone maintenance treatment and the production of time, space and subjects. *International Journal of Drug Policy, 17*(3), 192–202.

Fraser, S. (In press). Doing ontopolitically-oriented research: Synthesising concepts from the ontological turn for alcohol and other drug research and other social sciences. *International Journal of Drug Policy, 82.*

Fraser, S., & Moore, D. (2011a). Harm reduction and hepatitis C: On the ethics and politics of prevention and treatment. *Addiction Research and Theory, 19*(4), 375–379.

Fraser, S., & Moore, D. (2011b). *The drug effect: Health crime and society.* Melbourne: Cambridge University Press.

Fraser, S., Pienaar, K., Dilkes-Frayne, E., Moore, D., Kokanovic, R., Treloar, C., & Dunlop, A. (2017). Addiction stigma and the biopolitics of liberal modernity: A qualitative analysis. *International Journal of Drug Policy, 44*, 192–201.

Fraser, S., & Seear, K. (2011). *Making disease, making citizens: The politics of hepatitis C.* Aldershot: Ashgate.

Gane, E. (2014). Hepatitis C beware – The end is nigh. *The Lancet, 384*(9954), 1557–1560.

Hajarizadeh, B., Grebely, J., Martinello, M., Matthews, G., Lloyd, A., & Dore, G. (2016). Hepatitis C treatment as prevention: Evidence, feasibility, and challenges. *Lancet: Gastroenterology and Hepatology, 1*, 317–327.

Harris, M., Albers, E., & Swan, T. (2015). The promise of treatment as prevention for hepatitis C: Meeting the needs of people who inject drugs? *International Journal of Drug Policy, 26*, 963–969.

Hellard, M. (2014). Eliminating hepatitis C – an ambitious but achievable goal. *The Conversation.* March 28.

Hellard, M. D., Rolls, A., Sacks-Davis, R., Robins, G., Pattison, P., Higgs, P., … McBryde, E. (2014). The impact of injecting networks on hepatitis C transmission and treatment in people who inject drugs. *Hepatology, 60*(6), 1861–1870.

Hopwood, M., & Treloar, C. (2007). Pretreatment preparation and management of interferon-based therapy for hepatitis C virus infection. *Journal of Advanced Nursing, 59*(3), 248–254.

Johnson, J., & Lenton, E. (2017). *HIV and hepatitis pre- and post-test discussion in Victoria consultation report*. Melbourne: Australian Research Centre in Sex, Health and Society, La Trobe University.

Kracht, P. A. M., Arends, J. E., van Erpecum, K. J., Thijsen, S. F. T., Vlaminckx, B. J. M., Weersink, A. J. L., … Hoepelman, A. I. M. (2019). REtrieval And cure of Chronic Hepatitis C (REACH): results of micro-elimination in the Utrecht province. *Liver International, 39*(3), 455–462.

Lancaster, K., & Rhodes, T. (In press). Futuring a world without disease: Visualising the elimination of hepatitis C. *Critical Public Health*, 1–15.

Lancaster, K., Seear, K., & Ritter, A. (2018). *Reducing stigma and discrimination for people experiencing problematic alcohol and other drug use. Drug policy modelling program monograph series, 26*. Sydney: National Drug and Alcohol Research Centre.

Lazarus, J. V., Safreed-Harmon, K., Thursz, M. R., Dillon, J. F., El-Sayed, M. H., Elsharkawy, A. M., & Colombo, M. (2018). The micro-elimination approach to eliminating hepatitis C: Strategic and operational considerations. In *Seminars in liver disease* (Vol. 38, No. 03, pp. 181-192). Thieme Medical Publishers.

Lloyd, C. (2010). *Sinning and sinned against: The stigmatisation of problem drug users*. London: UK Drug Policy Commission.

MacLachlan, J. H., Smith, C., Towell, V., & Cowie, B. C. (2020). *Viral hepatitis mapping project: National report 2018–19*. Darlinghurst: Australasian Society for HIV, Viral Hepatitis and Sexual Health Medicine (ASHM). https://ashm.org.au/programs/Viral-Hepatitis-Mapping-Project/.

Madden, A., Hopwood, M., Neale, J., & Treloar, C. (2018a). Beyond cure: Patient reported outcomes of hepatitis C treatment among people who inject drugs in Australia. *Harm Reduction Journal, 15*(1), 1–8.

Madden, A., Hopwood, M., Neale, J., & Treloar, C. (2018b). Beyond interferon side effects: What residual barriers exist to DAA hepatitis C treatment for people who inject drugs? *PloS one, 13* (11), e0207226.

Malins, P. (2017). Desiring assemblages: A case for desire over pleasure in critical drug studies. *International Journal of Drug Policy, 49*, 126–132.

Martinello, M., Hajarizadeh, B., & Dore, G. J. (2018). Observations on the launch of new drugs for hepatitis C. *Australian Prescriber, 41*(1), 4.

Martinello, M., & Matthews, G. V. (2015). Enhancing the detection and management of acute hepatitis C virus infection. *International Journal of Drug Policy, 26*(10), 899–910.

Moore, D., & Fraser, S. (2006). Putting at risk what we know: Reflecting on the drug-using subject in harm reduction and its political implications. *Social Science and Medicine, 62*, 3035–3047.

Newman, C., MacGibbon, J., Smith, A. K., Broady, T., Lupton, D., Davis, M., & Holt, M. (2020). *Understanding trust in digital health among communities affected by BBVs and STIs in Australia*. Sydney: UNSW.

O'Kelly, M., Byrne, D., Naughten, E., Bergin, C., & Williams, C. (2016). Opt-out testing for blood-borne viruses in primary care: A multicentre, prospective study. *British Journal of General Practice, 66*(647), e392–e396.

Persson, A., Newman, C. E., Mao, L., & de Wit, J. (2016). On the margins of pharmaceutical citizenship: Not taking HIV medication in the "treatment revolution" era. *Medical Anthropology Quarterly, 30*(3), 359–377.

Prince, D. S., Pipicella, J. L., Fraser, M., Alvaro, F., Maley, M., Foo, H., & Levy, M. T. (2021). Screening emergency admissions at risk of chronic hepatitis C (SEARCH) to diagnose or 're-diagnose' infections is effective in Australia. *Journal of Viral Hepatitis, 28*(1), 121–128.

Rance, J., Rhodes, T., & Lancaster, K. (2021). Pharmaceutical citizenship in an era of universal access to hepatitis C treatment: Situated potentials and limits. *Health: An interdisciplinary journal for the social study of health, illness and medicine*. Early online.

Rhodes, T., & Treloar, C. (2008). The social production of hepatitis C risk among injecting drug users: A qualitative synthesis. *Addiction, 103*(10), 1593–1603.

Scott, N., Sacks-Davis, R., Wade, A. J., Stoove, M., Pedrana, A., Doyle, J. S., & Hellard, M. E. (2020). Australia needs to increase testing to achieve hepatitis C elimination. *Medical Journal of Australia, 212*(8), 365–370.

Seear, K., Fraser, S., Farrugia, A., & Valentine, K. (In press). Beyond a 'post-cure' world: Sketches for a new futurology of hepatitis C. *International Journal of Drug Policy*. Early online

Stoové, M., Wallace, J., Higgs, P., Pedrana, A., Goutzamanis, S., Latham, N., … Hellard, M. (2020). Treading lightly: Finding the best way to use public health surveillance of hepatitis C diagnoses to increase access to cure. *International Journal of Drug Policy, 75*, 102596.

Treloar, C., Rance, J., & Backmund, M. (2013). Understanding barriers to hepatitis C virus care and stigmatization from a social perspective. *Clinical Infectious Diseases, 57*(suppl_2), S51–S55.

Treloar, C., & Rhodes, T. (2009). The lived experience of hepatitis C and its treatment among injecting drug users: Qualitative synthesis. *Qualitative Health Research, 19*(9), 1321–1334.

Van Dijk, M., van Agt, F. M., & Drenth, J. P. H. (2020). Legal and ethical challenges in developing a Dutch nationwide hepatitis C retrieval project (CELINE). *International Journal of Health Policy Management, x*(x), 1–5.

Whiteley, D., Whittaker, A., Elliott, L., & Cunningham-Burley, S. (2018). Hepatitis C in a new therapeutic era: Recontextualising the lived experience. *Journal of Clinical Nursing, 27*(13-14), 2729–2739.

World Health Organization. (2016). *Combating hepatitis B and C to reach elimination by 2030*. Geneva: WHO.

World Health Organization. (2016). *Global health sector strategy on viral hepatitis: Towards ending viral hepatitis, 2016-2021*. Geneva: World Health Organization.

World Health Organization. (2017). *WHO guidelines on hepatitis B and C testing*. Geneva: World Health Organization.

Wright, C., Cogger, S., Hsieh, K., Goutzamanis, S., Hellard, M., & Higgs, P. (2019). "I'm obviously not dying so it's not something I need to sort out today": considering hepatitis C treatment in the era of direct acting antivirals. *Infection, Disease and Health, 24*(2), 58–66.

Making publics in a pandemic: Posthuman relationalities, 'viral' intimacies and COVID-19

Kiran Pienaar, Jacinthe Flore, Jennifer Power and Dean Murphy

ABSTRACT
The COVID-19 pandemic has placed sexual relationships into sharp focus as strict containment measures, including physical distancing and 'stay at home' restrictions, were initiated to control the spread of the virus. Governments in some jurisdictions prevented contact between non-cohabiting sexual partners (except for couples in pre-existing relationships), while community organisations recommended people avoid casual sexual encounters. This article analyses Australian media articles, commentary and public health messages published during March to October 2020 to explore the normative assumptions underpinning these measures. Applying posthumanist perspectives and Warner's (2002) conceptualisation of 'publics', we consider how COVID-19 public health advice enacts the (human) subject of public health as monogamous, coupled, and living with their partner or nuclear family. Those in non-normative relationships and households are not only excluded from this narrow enactment of the 'ideal' public health subject, but are rendered potentially risky disease vectors by virtue of their alternative kinship arrangements. We explore the implications of these findings for the more-than-human relationalities that shape health inequalities and processes of marginalisation during public health crises, and we offer suggestions for public health measures that address the needs of diverse 'publics'.

Introduction

The COVID-19 (coronavirus) pandemic placed sexual, familial and intimate relationships into sharp relief as governments across the world introduced strict measures ('lockdowns') to control the spread of the virus. These included physical distancing and 'stay at home' restrictions aimed at limiting physical contact to members of one's immediate household. Governments in some jurisdictions prevented contact between non-cohabiting sexual partners (except for couples in pre-existing intimate relationships), while community organisations recommended people limit casual sexual encounters and 'non-essential' socialising. This article critically analyses COVID-19 public health discourses in Australia to shed light on their implicit assumptions about the relationship between viral containment, intimacy and private domestic space. Our analysis examines Australian public health messages, media articles and commentary published during the first and second waves of the pandemic (March to October 2020) to explore the definitions of 'home', 'household' and 'family' underpinning physical distancing measures.

With a total of 32,129 cumulative COVID-19 cases at the time of writing (Australian Government Department of Health, 20 July 2021), Australia has not been immune from the effects of the pandemic. However, its impacts have been disproportionately felt in the state of Victoria (BBC News, 2020) which has accounted for over two-thirds of cases (despite representing only around one-quarter of Australia's overall population). As other Australian states and territories returned to normal activities with some restrictions in mid-May 2020, Victoria experienced a rapid rise in COVID-19 cases in June. As a result, a second round of restrictions was introduced targeting various 'hotspots' in Victoria. By July, these restrictions were broadened and a second lockdown was introduced for metropolitan Melbourne and one adjacent local government area. Despite these measures, infection rates continued to rise and in early August 2020, the Victorian Premier declared a state of disaster, imposing tighter restrictions on affected areas. These included a nightly curfew for six weeks and a five-kilometre radius limit on movement, with substantial fines enforceable for anyone breaching the restrictions.

Importantly for our purposes, the restrictions had significant implications for households, those in intimate relationships, families and single people living alone. While non-cohabiting couples were able to visit each other, single people living alone could not see friends or family. Following public debate on the plight of the half a million Victorians who live alone (Visontay, 2020) and an online petition calling for social bubbles for single people (Ford, 2020), the government eventually introduced 'single-person bubbles' in mid-September. This measure allowed people who live alone to nominate one person as their social contact for the duration of the restrictions. Single people could not nominate an entire household (defined as more than one person living in a single dwelling) and when visiting their 'bubble partner's' dwelling, no other adult was permitted to be present for the duration of the visit. Furthermore, those in a single bubble were required to wear face masks while visiting, a measure that the state's Chief Health Officer later conceded was not practical (Mitchell, 2020) and, importantly, one that did not apply to non-cohabiting intimate partners. As we go on to show, such restrictions are not only impractical, they also rely on normative assumptions that warrant interrogation.

To examine these assumptions, we draw on the concept of posthumanist performativity (Barad, 2003) and critical scholarship on 'publics' and 'counterpublics' (Warner, 2002). In doing so, we consider how COVID-19 public health advice enacts the (human) subject of public health as monogamous, coupled and living with their partner or nuclear family in a hetero- or homonormative kinship model. Those in non-normative kinship structures, including blended or extended families, chosen families (Weston, 1997), non-cohabiting couples, polyamorous people and single parents, are both excluded from this narrow enactment of the 'ideal' public health subject, and implicitly rendered potentially risky disease vectors by virtue of their alternative kinship arrangements. In posthumanist terms, our analysis suggests that the 'public' of public health is constituted narrowly to exclude those whose kinship structures do not fit conventional definitions, rendering them less-than-fully-human abject Others who may undermine efforts to contain the pandemic. We explore the implications of these findings for the more-than-human relationalities that shape health inequalities and processes of marginalisation during public health crises. Inspired by recent feminist and posthumanist scholarship, we argue that the pandemic presents an opportunity for rethinking dominant logics of care to redress, rather than reinforce, the persistent inequalities dividing our societies.

Background

As the COVID-19 pandemic unfolds, researchers have devoted attention to its sociopolitical dimensions and the far-reaching social changes it has wrought. In a recent special issue of this journal on 'sociology and the COVID-19 pandemic', Rahman (2020) traces how India's efforts to contain the pandemic have entrenched discrimination against poor people and ethnic minorities due in part to the legacy of India's caste system. Consistent with the focus on the relationship between the pandemic and social inequalities, Goggin and Ellis (2020) highlight how COVID-19 responses have overlooked people with disabilities. Critical drug research similarly highlights the tensions between COVID-19 containment measures and the precarity of people who use drugs (e.g. Chang, Agliata, & Guarinieri, 2020) with some scholars arguing that physical distancing measures require people who consume drugs to 'choose between avoidance of COVID-19 and the intimacies of drug use that contribute to their survival' (Schlosser & Harris, 2020, p. 102896). Read together, these critical analyses offer valuable insights into the ways in which vulnerable communities are disproportionately affected by COVID-19. However, empirical research to date has yet to examine the assumptions underpinning coronavirus containment measures and their implications for minorities and marginalised groups, which is the focus of our analysis.

Given this focus, a second relevant strand of research addresses COVID's impact on minorities and its implications for intimacy. Drawing on their expertise in sexology and psychology, Dewitte, Otten, and Walker (2020), for example, present interviews with three specialists in sexology and psychology to discuss the effects of lockdown on sex and intimacy. The discussion mostly centres on co-habiting, heterosexual couples, as illustrated by the following advice from one of the experts interviewed: '[I]f you are able to set up some private time, get the children settled with snacks and a movie, or wake up before they get up in the morning, you might want to try something new. Crack out some sexual toys, find a blindfold, try a new position, or act out a sexual fantasy' (Dewitte et al., 2020, p. 548). Not only does this suggestion assume a heterosexual, middle-class, nuclear family with a stable job and housing, it also uncritically presents individual solutions to the challenges of intimacy during lockdown, overlooking the structural and social factors that affect intimacy. Importantly, the exclusionary norms at work in public health measures and their implications for people outside the normative nuclear family remain unquestioned.

Prompted by the limitations of such approaches, we turn to two essays on the impact of coronavirus restrictions on the governance of sex and intimacy. The first by McKenzie (2020) argues that the Australian federal government's response presumed widespread coupledom, ignoring the needs of single people or those living alone. Moreover, McKenzie notes that official discourses on physical distancing regulations were 'strangely sexless' and did not publicly acknowledge the implications of the restrictions for sex and intimacy (McKenzie, 2020, p. 11). The second piece by Thorneycroft and Nicholas (2021) applies queer and crip theories to critique individualising conceptions of coronavirus risk. Focussing on the implications for queer sexual practices during the pandemic, they argue that this contemporary moment 'allows for a reconceptualising of responsibility and ethical sex away from their pervasive normative foundations, towards instead a (queer) sexual ethics focused on pleasure' (Thorneycroft & Nicholas, 2021, p. 104). Rather than centring sexual risk and responsibility, such an ethics, they suggest, is attentive to non-normative modes of intimacy and care. This queer rethinking of sex and intimacy in the context of COVID-19 offers valuable insights for our efforts to interrogate the normative assumptions governing viral containment measures. To interpret the relationship between these social norms and the 'human' subjects of public health, we turn to the theoretical literatures on posthumanism and the production of publics.

Posthumanist performativity and the making of publics

To explore how the human subject of public health is differentially constituted in discourses on COVID-19, we draw on feminist theorist Karen Barad's (2003; 2007) 'posthumanist performativity'. Her approach is informed by feminist post-structuralist theories, notably Butler's (1999) theory of gender performativity, which disrupts the sex/gender binary by refiguring gender as an iterative effect of discourse. While Barad acknowledges the contribution of Butler's approach, she argues that it neglects to account for precisely how discursive practices constitute material bodies. In proposing the concept of posthumanist performativity, she aims to 'sharpen the theoretical tool of performativity' to account for the agency of matter in constituting realities (2003, p. 803). Importantly, and in contrast to conventional approaches that seek to identify the discrete effects of material or discursive factors, posthumanist performativity recognises the 'conjoined material-discursive nature' of the practices that produce realities (Barad, 2007, p. 152).

Implicit here is the recognition that performativity is not the sole prerogative of humans. Techno-scientific and other 'non-human' practices and relations also have agency to materialise realities. By challenging the anthropocentric assumptions associated with poststructuralist conceptions of performativity, Barad's account reconstitutes the boundary between the human and non-human as dynamic and emergent, rather than fixed and naturally given. This rethinking is particularly useful for our analysis as it disrupts the assumption that the human subject of public health pre-exists public health discourses. Instead by treating the human of public health as constituted, in part, through particular health practices and injunctions, this approach allows us to trace the co-production of the human and the ideal public health subject. We explore this co-construction as a means of probing the performative work of COVID public health discourses, tracking how the human subject of public health is narrowly constituted to exclude marginalised groups, in the process entrenching their precarity. In doing so, we treat public health discourses, not as representations of a prior reality, but as material-discursive enactments that produce particular realities and health subjects.

Our analysis is also informed by Michael Warner's (2002) influential account of the production of publics. According to Warner, public discourse does not simply address a pre-existing public, but calls particular publics into being:

> Public discourse says not only 'Let a public exist' but 'Let it have this character, speak this way, see the world in this way'. It then goes in search of confirmation that such a public exists, with greater or lesser success – success being further attempts to cite, circulate, and realize the world understanding it articulates (2002, p. 422).

Crucial here is the performative role of discourse in giving publics a particular shape and character. In other words, the production of publics is not a straightforward, top-down process in which individuals are simply grouped into publics and then begin to act accordingly. Rather, publics materialise through specific discursive practices and as such they are open to change and contestation.

Recent critical scholarship has applied these ideas across different policy domains to consider how public policy constructs stratified publics, reinforcing the social privilege of some groups while marginalising others (for example, in relation to drug policy, Farrugia & Fraser, 2017; and in the context of sex education, Rasmussen & Leahy, 2018). Attentive to power dynamics and processes of marginalisation, this work tracks the performative effects of public discourses in producing dominant publics and counterpublics. The term counterpublics was first coined by Nancy Fraser (1990) to highlight the social groups excluded by the dominant public sphere who form competing, subaltern publics. As Fraser puts it, counterpublics 'mark themselves off unmistakably from any general or dominant public' (1990, pp. 84–89). Challenging the assumption of a single, unitary public, the notion of counterpublics articulates the diverse, conflicting publics produced in public discourses. Especially relevant to our work is the concept of 'counter-public health', proposed by Kane Race (2009, 2010) to critique moralised notions of health and examine how 'political investment in a particular idea of public membership (e.g. family values, a drug-free nation, etc.) thwarts rational responses to public health' (Race, 2010, para. 3). Applying these ideas to coronavirus containment measures, we consider the publics produced by these measures and their role in reinforcing inequalities and processes of marginalisation during public health crises.

Method

This article presents a case study of the public health response to COVID-19 in Australia, with a particular focus on Victoria, Australia's worst-affected state accounting for more than 90% of COVID deaths in the second wave and having experienced the most severe and protracted COVID restrictions (BBC News, 2020). Our analysis draws on COVID-related public health advice, commentary and news media articles, published between 1 March to 26 October 2020, coinciding with the first and second waves of the pandemic in Australia with 26 October marking the lifting of stage 4 restrictions in metropolitan Melbourne. Using the search terms 'COVID-19 restrictions', 'lockdown Victoria/Melbourne' 'single bubble', 'public housing lockdown', 'COVID-19, intimacy and sex', we conducted Google searches for this date range which yielded over 500 sources. We excluded any material that did not address the COVID restrictions directly (e.g. general news articles on the pandemic). This generated a corpus of 38 media articles, 23 commentaries and 22 public health messages from government bodies and community organisations. While most of the media articles and commentary are by Australian outlets, we also included relevant international material addressing the implications of containment measures for disadvantaged groups, minorities and those in non-normative intimate or familial relationships. This enabled us to place Australia's COVID-19 response in a broader international context and to identify more inclusive public health approaches to containing the pandemic.

We recognise that in composing a corpus for analysis we are implicated in the process of producing publics and counterpublics. A different dataset or even the same one informed by other analytic concerns would have materialised different health publics and counterpublics. Indeed, our point is that, far from being and fixed and stable, publics emerge through specific discursive-material practices, including those associated with the research processes. In Barad's terms, these practices are performative: they call publics into being. Thus, when particular practices change, so too do the contours and character of the mutually constituted publics. Our concern then is to trace the specificities of the publics produced through Victoria's COVID measures and community counter-responses, focussing on the exclusions these practices generate and, in the case of the counter-responses, the exclusions they seek to challenge in relation to dominant forms of kinship, sex and intimacy.

The data were coded thematically using an iterative inductive approach in which a preliminary list of codes was drawn up based on our overarching interest in the assumptions and subjectification effects of COVID-19 public health advice. The coding frame was informed by the relevant literatures on the sociology of pandemics, the construction of publics and their implications for the subjects of public health. The codes were tested on a sub-set of data by the first author, and the coding frame was then refined: supplementary codes were added across the dataset to capture a wider range of themes derived from the empirical material (Dicks, 2012). Codes relating to the Victorian restrictions (particularly regarding physical distancing and stay-at-home measures; visiting intimate partners, family and friends; and social gatherings) were reviewed to reveal three recurring themes in the data: 1) the directive to 'stay home, stay safe'; 2) the governance of sex, intimacy and social connection via the lockdown measures; and 3) community resistance and counter-responses to these measures. These themes guided the analysis in terms of the subjects of public health that they enact, the exclusions and health inequalities they produce, and modes of resistance to these exclusionary health publics (or what we call 'queer counterpublics'). Focussing on marginalised communities, single people and those in non-normative relationships, our analysis highlights how Australia's COVID-19 response has reinscribed the middle class, nuclear family as the basic unit of social life.

Analysis

'Stay home, stay safe: we're all in this together'

At the centre of the Australian government's COVID-19 response was the directive to 'stay home, stay safe', followed by the slogan 'we're all in this together' (North Western Melbourne Primary Health Network, 2020). This message was delivered in sombre tones by government officials such as the Victorian Premier, Daniel Andrews, who warned of COVID-19 mortality risks and exhorted Victorians to 'Stay home. Save lives'. As he stressed, 'Saving lives is everyone's job [...] This is about all of us and unless you want to be burying an elderly relative or your best mate or your parents [...]

then do the right thing. *It's very, very simple. Stay at home*' (Andrews, 2020, emphasis added). While these messages may appear uncontroversial and centred on solidarity and inclusivity, they contain a number of assumptions about access to private, domestic space that warrant scrutiny. For example, as scholars have noted, home is neither equally accessible nor a safe space for many, including those experiencing gendered domestic or family violence (Kay, 2020), many LGBTIQ people including those affected by homo/transphobic family violence with trans and gender diverse young people disproportionately affected (Byron, Robinson, Davies, & D'Souza, 2021), and those who are homeless or sleeping rough (Casey & Mohan, 2020). In relation to those experiencing homelessness, it is worth noting that in the first wave of the pandemic, the Victorian and New South Wales' state governments accommodated homeless people in hotels, suggesting awareness of their plight under COVID restrictions. However, these support measures were short-lived with funding running out after a few months leaving those affected once again at risk of homelessness (Gearin, 2020). Other vulnerable populations who could not comply with the directive to stay home include people in prisons, detention centres and refugee camps, as well as people in residential aged care facilities, as starkly highlighted by the number of infections and deaths in Victorian aged care centres (Cousins, 2020). In short, staying home is not as 'simple' as government officials claim. For many marginalised groups, home is associated with 'precarity, violence and terror, either because the lack of a materially stable home, or because of the violence contained within it, or both' (Kay, 2020, p. 887).

Feminist writer, Sophie Lewis offers a trenchant critique of the assumptions implicit in 'stay at home' directives:

> 'Staying home' is what is somehow self-evidently supposed to keep us well. But there are several problems with this [...] problems one might summarize as the mystification of the couple-form; the romanticisation of kinship; and the sanitization of the fundamentally unsafe space that is private property [...] Such standard homes are where, after all, everyone secretly knows the majority of earthly violence goes down (Lewis, 2020, para. 2).

Therefore, while we recognise the importance of isolation measures to contain the spread of the virus, we follow the lead of Lewis and other feminist scholars in highlighting the normative assumptions built into official pandemic responses (e.g. Kay, 2020; Ticktin, 2020). Made in the name of public health, these injunctions naturalise the home as an apolitical place of refuge and safety, and in the process, they efface the constitutive exclusions of the 'dominant health public'. We would do well to ask: how do you stay at home when you are homeless? Or where do you go when home is not safe? We suggest that uncritical acceptance of stay-at-home directives risks reinforcing the myth of 'home-as-haven', effacing the gender, race and class structures that shape access to a safe, private home.

The impact of restrictions on vulnerable communities was perhaps most strikingly evidenced in the government's response to the rise in coronavirus cases in several Melbourne public housing complexes. With little warning, Victorian authorities locked down the housing blocks, and residents were subjected to a heavy police presence and severe restrictions not imposed in outbreaks in more affluent areas (HRW, 2020). Many public housing residents are from low socioeconomic or migrant backgrounds and the restrictions drew criticism from the Victorian Public Tenants Association for stigmatising already vulnerable communities (Weedon, 2020). Indeed, Victoria's ombudsman later found that the lockdown violated human rights laws and called for the government to apologise to residents, but government officials refused, maintaining that they acted in the best interests of the community to save lives (Boseley, 2020). However, some residents commented that the strict lockdown made them feel like criminals and entrenched the existing vulnerabilities of lower-income groups and ethnic minorities (Om, 2020). For example, a Somali resident suggested that 'the enforced lockdown is a direct reflection of the systematic inequalities [people face] in public housing' (Anisa cited in Carrasco, Faleh, & Dangol, 2020, para. 6). Another resident raised concern about the lockdown's impact on migrant residents with experience of trauma and persecution in their countries of origin: 'This community is made up of many people who have fled war, who have complicated mental health issues, whose families have been racially profiled and targeted by police' (Iman cited in Carrasco et al., 2020, para. 6). These comments point to the disproportionate impact of restrictions on vulnerable communities.

The response to the COVID-19 outbreak in Melbourne's public housing blocks also points to the ideal 'home' that is enacted in public health discourse: a large, suburban, privately owned house with multiple bedrooms and outdoor space, not a public, high-rise apartment in the inner city. By extension, the ideal household is assumed to comprise only the nuclear family with each member having their own bedroom. Households consisting of multiple generations and/or extended family living in a small, overcrowded space and sharing facilities is the antithesis of the 'normative Australian household' assumed in COVID-19 containment measures. As the government's response to the outbreak in public housing blocks shows, such households are treated as a risk to public health. The idealised notion of 'home' and family underpinning public health discourses suggests a need to critically examine the logic governing pandemic responses, and in particular what is elided by blithe expressions claiming, 'we're all in this together'. In posthumanist performative terms, we argue that insofar as the prescribed pandemic response compromises the most marginalised in our societies, it effectively renders these populations lesser humans with expendable rights. In other words, public health measures are performative in that they produce stratified health publics, entrenching the privilege of some groups and disadvantaging others. In the case of COVID-19, the directive to 'stay home' as the undifferentiated, dominant prophylactic response has reinforced the precarity of marginalised communities, including homeless people, poor and culturally diverse communities, people in prison and detention centres, and those in residential care facilities (including aged care, disability care and drug treatment centres). Linked to the ideal household implicit in stay-home restrictions are normative assumptions privileging the couple or nuclear family as the basic social unit. In what follows, we explore these assumptions and their implications for the governance of intimacy and social relations.

Couple normativity and the 'single social bubble'

As mentioned above, the Australian federal government's COVID-19 response comprised restrictions on social interactions, including physical distancing measures and strict two-person limits on social gatherings with exceptions for people in the same household. The measures had significant implications for the governance of sex, intimacy and social connection, and their impact varied according to people's living arrangements and relationship status. While non-cohabiting couples were able to visit each other, single people living alone could not visit friends or family. Further compounding the physical isolation was the imposition of a travel rule during the intensified lockdown in Melbourne from July to October, which prevented residents (with few exceptions, such as non-cohabiting, intimate partners) from travelling more than five kilometres from their home. Like other physical distancing measures, this restriction presumes that most people live in households comprising normative, nuclear families or couples. Not only does the enforced isolation disadvantage single people living far from friends and family, it also overlooks that 521,828 Victorians live on their own and the number of solo households is growing (Taylor, 2020). The indefinite isolation took a toll, with one Melbourne mental health service reporting high levels of anxiety among single people living alone (Asher, 2020). The yearning for touch and physical connection is apparent in accounts from Melbourne residents living alone: 'How am I going to deal with this, where do you get that physical connection [...]? Normally you'd go out and have a hug with a friend, but now we're not supposed to do anything' (Lindberg cited in Asher, 2020, n.p.).

By allowing visits between intimate partners on the grounds that they constitute modes of 'care' and 'support', Australia's coronavirus restrictions implicitly renounced other kinds of care including those associated with queer forms of kinship, close friendships and casual sexual practices: 'Permitting visits to partners for 'care'-based reasons demonstrates an implicit abjection and disavowal of other modes of sexual relationality, and potentially the ongoing taboo around discussing sexuality as a need or sexual pleasure in official discourses, with risk once again dominating sexuality discourse' (Thorneycroft & Nicholas, 2021, p. 106). The focus of policy and media discourses centred on health and well-being with visits between non-cohabiting partners justified for mental health reasons (Costa, 2020). Indeed, mention of sex was conspicuously absent in official discourses despite the implications of the regulations for physical touch and intimacy (McKenzie, 2020). In contrast to Australia's response, governments in other jurisdictions took a more open, pragmatic approach to sex in the context of COVID-19: the Dutch government explicitly encouraged single residents to find a trusted '*seksbuddy*' and Danish health authorities expressed support for casual sexual encounters (Boffey, 2020).

In addition to omitting any reference to sex and intimacy in relation to COVID-19, Australia's restrictions produce a hegemonic public normatively defined as consisting of middle-class, nuclear families or couples. Other scholars have likewise observed the privileging of 'coupledom' during the COVID-19 pandemic and highlighted its exclusionary effects. For example, Roseneil refers to the 'tyranny of coupledom' noting:

> the Covid-19 pandemic has seen a significant intensification of the couple norm, and it highlights in new ways the stigma and marginalisation faced by those who are not conventionally coupled. Lockdowns forcibly redomesticate sexual and intimate life, cutting off physical connection between people who do not cohabit (2020, para. 6).

In a similar critique of official stay-at-home directives, Fitzgerald observes:

> Here, the reproductive legacy of epidemiology, a discipline centred on the health and viability of a certain idea of population, reaches a kind of logical endpoint through the deployment of heteronormative and middle-class homemaking [...] The reproductive family unit [...] hygienically separated in its new-build home, with easy road access to a large supermarket – this is the infrastructural vision of a newly suburbanized epidemiology (2020, para. 10).

In official discourses, this intimate public (Berlant, 1998) is legitimised as necessary to contain the spread of the virus and 'save lives'. As Victorian Premier, Daniel Andrews emphasised, 'Stay. In. Your. House [...] Do not have guests over [...] Do not leave home unless it's absolutely necessary [...] Saving lives is everyone's job' (Andrews, 2020). It is hard to argue with this logic and it works here as a powerful authorising move that obscures the social norms informing public health practices. In other words, the seemingly unassailable imperative to prevent the spread of disease effectively inoculates normative public health practices from critique, rendering them self-evidently 'good'.

Yet despite the apparently incontrovertible status of viral containment measures, pockets of resistance emerged at the margins. For example, following public debate on the plight of Victorians who live alone (Visontay, 2020) and an online petition calling for social bubbles for single people (Ford, 2020), the government introduced 'single-person bubbles' in mid-September. Such sites of resistance to the dominant public enacted in COVID-19 restrictions can be understood as counterpublics in that they position themselves as distinct from the mythical 'general' public of public health. In this respect, Ford's petition argued that the restrictions discriminated against those without an intimate partner and called for the government to recognise that 'single people have as much right to social connection as intimate partners' (Ford, 2020). These counterpublics challenge the redomestication of social and intimate life in the name of public health, and demand state recognition of solo households and networks of care and intimacy beyond the nuclear family. As we discuss in the next section, queer communities also emerged as a site of resistance (or counterpublic) that sought to unsettle the normative values and social relations enacted via COVID public health restrictions.

Queer counterpublics: LGBTIQ community organisations' responses to the pandemic

While government directives in response to COVID-19 overlooked care practices beyond the hetero- or homonormative[1] nuclear family, Australian community and sexual health bodies eventually began to address them explicitly by considering the implications of physical distancing measures for sex, intimacy and connection. Although messaging early in the pandemic advised LGBTIQ communities to avoid all sex with casual partners (and advocated restricting sex to co-habiting partners), by mid-2020 these bodies began to promote harm reduction strategies for reducing the risk of infection while having causal sex. In June 2020 the Australasian Society for HIV, Viral Hepatitis and Sexual Health Medicine (AHSM) released a statement endorsing a harm reduction approach to casual sex during the pandemic. Informed by consultations with local community-based organisations such as ACON (Australia's largest LGBTIQ and HIV service organisation), and the Scarlet Alliance (Australia's sex worker organisation), this approach advocates sexual practices that may reduce the risk of coronavirus transmission (e.g. contactless sex, masturbation, online encounters, sexting, avoiding positions that involve face-to-face contact, washing before/after sex) (AHSM Taskforce on BBVs, 2020). Similarly, Victorian LGBTIQ organisation, Thorne Harbour Health (THH), released a consumer information sheet offering pragmatic advice on casual sex during the pandemic:

> If you and a regular casual partner (aka a fuck buddy) are both practicing physical distancing from others, you can have sex with one another with a low risk of acquiring COVID-19. However, communication is key. You need to have a clear and honest conversation about what exposure each of you has to others at this time. You also need to let each other know immediately if either of you becomes unwell (THH, 2020).

This pragmatism is also evident in LGBTIQ organisations' acknowledgement of non-monogamous sexual relationships:

> You may be in a monogamous, polyamorous or any other exclusive relationship with one or more people and choose to continue to have sex together. Whether you live with them or not [...] there is still a risk of one of you unknowingly coming into contact with the virus outside your home and then bringing it into the household. Talk to each other, assess your situation and make that decision together (ACON, 2020).

These responses are informed by the legacy of HIV activism in response to mainstream HIV responses which often sought to shut down discussions of sex and pleasure, placing abstinence or monogamy at the centre of prevention messages. In contrast, queer community responses foregrounded fun, pleasure and eroticism – creating counterpublic discourses on non-monogamy, group sex, anal sex and use of illicit drugs. This was not done to deliberately transgress normative public health discourses but rather as part of an ethic of care that brings ideas about safe sex into sexual practices and cultures. As mentioned earlier, Race has drawn on Warner's concept of counterpublics to describe community responses to HIV as forms of counterpublic health:

> As a concept, [counterpublic health] tries to get a handle on some of the dynamics that impede the formulation of practical strategies of care within such populations [queers, women, and drug users], highlighting the sense in which these dangers are a function, in part, of hegemonic norms (2009, p. 162).

Therefore, rather than trying to disavow queer sexuality and enact punitive public health responses that foreclose sex, counterpublic health treats queer sexual practices and cultures as crucial to effective public health responses.

In the cases of both HIV and COVID-19, the advice offered by LGBTIQ organisations recognises the social significance of non-monogamous sexual relationships in queer communities and in doing so legitimises queer forms of sociality. Moreover, and in contrast to some of the government messaging, the health promotion messages of these organisations are unifying and inclusive of diverse relationships and sexual practices. Evoking the history of the HIV crisis and the queer support systems that emerged in response, Thorne Harbour Health's information sheet closes with the following advice:

> Keep kind and carry on. Obviously, this is not the first time our community has faced a health issue that has impacted our sexual pleasure and wellbeing. We are incredibly good at adopting effective health strategies – and that will be true of COVID-19. Let's look out for ourselves and each other in a difficult time (THH, 2020).

These examples suggest that those excluded from the dominant health public are finding innovative ways of creating more inclusive forms of connection and care. Extending Berlant's (1998) concept of 'intimate publics' we refer to these alternative care networks as 'intimate counterpublics'. Inspired by their inclusive ethos, we conclude with some reflections on how we might build on these efforts to counter the exclusionary effects of some public health measures.

Conclusion: Towards a posthumanist ethics of care

While Australia's coronavirus response has been effective in containing the virus, it has not been without problems. Indeed, as we have shown, Australia's model has relied on several normative assumptions that performatively constitute a 'health public' narrowly defined to exclude marginalised groups, including poor communities, culturally and linguistically diverse groups, homeless people, and those in non-traditional household structures (e.g. single people, blended families, multi-generation households). We are, of course, not trying to diminish the importance of viral containment measures but rather seeking to highlight their exclusionary assumptions and implications for marginalised publics. Our analysis reveals how COVID-19 public health measures are anchored in processes of normalisation that work to produce nuclear households as the dominant public. In doing so, they elevate heteronormative, romantic relationships above any other kind of relationships, including companionate friendships, platonic partnerships, blended families and queer forms of kinship. Of course, in many ways, it is unsurprising that coronavirus containment measures are deeply normative and exclusionary as scholars have long critiqued the exclusionary effects of public health practices particularly in relation to sexual minorities (e.g. Warner, 1999). In her classic piece, Rubin (1984) observed the ways in which some types of sex (e.g. casual, queer sex) are pathologised while others (usually heteronormative, monogamous sex) are valorised. In the context of COVID-19 restrictions, we see that contemporary public health measures are not immune from reproducing heteronormativity and other exclusionary social norms, such as the 'couple norm' and economic privilege. Such measures are part of a constellation of practices and institutions that centre the middle-class, nuclear family as the foundational unit of social membership.

Given the potential of pandemic responses to amplify existing social inequalities, we argue that the pandemic presents an opportunity to disrupt dominant logics and infrastructures of care. Against utilitarian, rationalist models that privilege the human as the subject and object of care, we posit care as a collective endeavour distributed across the human/non-human spectrum. On this rethinking, care is not the unique, feminised prerogative of individual human subjects but is a shared practice vital to the 'flourishing of humans and non-human life' (Chatzidakas et al., 2020, p. 893). Calling for a feminist ethics of care in response to COVID-19, disability scholars Fietz, Guedes de Mello, and Fonseca (2020, para. 11) write: 'Thinking with care presumes looking at contexts that include different people and families, many of whose living conditions are not easily adapted to social distancing. Covid-19 [...] forces us to live in a situation of constant tension and open-ended futures that render reflections and discussions on care practices ever more urgent'. To this we would add that adopting a feminist ethics of care entails the development of public health approaches responsive to the needs of diverse publics, including 'intimate counterpublics' and all those who are otherwise marginalised or effaced in dominant public discourses. As we have seen, these diverse publics include homeless people, aged care residents, survivors of domestic violence, and those in non-traditional households such as blended families, queer chosen families and single people living alone.

In advocating for an alternative ethics of care inspired by feminist, posthumanist scholarship, it is important to recognise the care practices that consumers and community organisations are already enacting, and their role in producing intimate counterpublics. As we have highlighted, LGBTIQ organisations in Australia have recognised the need for inclusive pandemic responses that address care and connection, alongside prevention and containment strategies. The New Zealand government's response is also noteworthy in this regard: its key message, 'be kind' centers compassion and empathy as guiding principles governing the pandemic response. Not only was New Zealand the first country to introduce support bubbles, its public health messaging encouraged New Zealanders to look out for the vulnerable in their communities. As one UK commentator put it in reflecting on the lessons this approach offers to other countries grappling with the effects of COVID-19, 'If New Zealand teaches us anything, it's […] that an ethic of support, compassion and mutual understanding will be key to living well in the coming months' (Long, 2020, para. 13). Importantly, such care practices extend beyond the nuclear family, challenging its status as the normative social unit. These alternative kinship structures and the logics of care they enact are not unlike the forms of kinship that queer people have created based on affective ties or shared needs, rather than biogenetics (Weston, 1997). As Ticktin (2020, para. 23) notes, 'COVID has generated the need for new relationships with friends, comrades, neighbors, coparents, lovers and ex-lovers — relationships that require deeper trust and sharing in new, respectful ways that limit exposure to risk, while still enabling sociality'. There is much to be learnt from the creative responses of those working to ensure that coronavirus containment measures address the needs of the most marginalised, whose precarity otherwise risks being reinforced by the pandemic.

Note

1. Australia's stay-home restrictions can be read as inclusive of homonormative forms of kinship that broadly align with heteronuclear models. However, as we go on to show the restrictions exclude relationship and kinship practices that do not conform to this normative model, including casual sexual partnerships, companionate friendships and queer chosen families.

Disclosure statement

No potential conflict of interest was reported by the authors.

ORCID

Kiran Pienaar http://orcid.org/0000-0003-4770-7882
Jacinthe Flore http://orcid.org/0000-0002-3136-9236
Jennifer Power http://orcid.org/0000-0002-6566-3214
Dean Murphy http://orcid.org/0000-0003-2752-7091

References

ACON. (2020). COVID-19 and our communities. (9 October). Retrieved from https://www.acon.org.au/what-we-are-here-for/covid19/#sex-in-the-era-of-covid-19.

AHSM Taskforce on BBVs. (2020). ASHM COVID-19 Taskforce recommendations to clinicians and healthcare workers on harm reduction approaches to casual sex during the COVID-19 pandemic. Retrieved from https://ashm.org.au/covid-19/clinical-care/harm-minimisation-approaches-to-casual-sex/.

Andrews, D. (2020). Stay home, save lives. Retrieved from https://www.facebook.com/watch/?v=218306979422749.

Asher, N. (2020). Coronavirus isolation measures taking toll on people who live alone. *ABC News* (1 April). Retrieved from https://www.abc.net.au/news/2020-04-01/coronavirus-self-isolation-measures-causing-loneliness/12107884.

Barad, K. (2003). Posthumanist performativity: Toward an understanding of how matter comes to matter. *Signs: Journal of Women in Culture and Society, 28*(3), 801–831.

Barad, K. (2007). *Meeting the universe halfway: Quantum physics and the entanglement of matter and meaning.* Durham: Duke University Press.

BBC News. (2020). Covid in Australia: Melbourne to exit 112-day lockdown. *BBC News Australia* (27 October). Retrieved from https://www.bbc.com/news/world-australia-54686812.

Berlant, L. (1998). Intimacy: A special issue. *Critical Inquiry, 24*(2), 281–288. Retrieved from http://www.jstor.org/stable/1344169.

Boffey, D. (2020). Dutch official advice to single people: find a sex buddy for lockdown. *The Guardian* (16 May). Retrieved from https://www.theguardian.com/world/2020/may/15/dutch-official-advice-to-single-people-find-a-sex-buddy-for-lockdown-coronavirus.

Boseley, M. (2020). Melbourne public housing Covid lockdown violated human rights, Victoria's ombudsman finds. *The Guardian* (17 December). Retrieved from https://www.theguardian.com/australia-news/2020/dec/17/melbourne-public-housing-covid-lockdown-violated-human-rights-victorias-ombudsman-finds.

Butler, J. (1999). *Gender trouble: Feminism and the subversion of identity.* London: Routledge.

Byron, P., Robinson, K., Davies, C., & D'Souza, S. (2021). *LGBTQ+ young people, COVID-19, & service provision in Australia: A Twenty10 case study.* Sydney: University of Technology Sydney.

Carrasco, S., Faleh, M., & Dangol, N. (2020). Our lives matter – Melbourne public housing residents talk about why COVID-19 hits them hard. *The Conversation* (24 July). Retrieved from https://theconversation.com/our-lives-matter-melbourne-public-housing-residents-talk-about-why-covid-19-hits-them-hard-142901.

Casey, L., & Mohan, N. (2020). It's taken the coronavirus crisis for people to see rough sleeping for the public health emergency it is. *The Policy Institute* (6 April 2020).

Chang, J., Agliata, J., & Guarinieri, M. (2020). COVID-19 – enacting a 'new normal' for people who use drugs. *International Journal of Drug Policy, 83*, 102832. doi:10.1016/j.drugpo.2020.102832

Chatzidakis, A., Hakim, J., Littler, J., Rottenberg, C., & Segal, L. (2020). From carewashing to radical care: the discursive explosions of care during Covid-19. *Feminist Media Studies 20*(6), 889–895.

Costa, J. (2020). Intimate personal relationship visits OK under Victoria's lockdown, but managing it a bit grey. ABC News (17 August). Retrieved from https://www.abc.net.au/news/2020-08-17/managing-love-and-relationships-in-coronavirus-lockdown/1256058.

Cousins, S. (2020). Experts criticise Australia's aged care failings over COVID-19. *The Lancet, 396* (10259), 1322–1323. doi:10.1016/S0140-6736(20)32206-6

Dewitte, M., Otten, C., & Walker, L. (2020). Making love in the time of corona – Considering relationships in lockdown. *Nature Reviews Urology, 17*(10), 547–553. doi:10.1038/s41585-020-0365-1

Dicks, B. (2012). *Digital qualitative research methods.* London: SAGE Publications.

Farrugia, A., & Fraser, S. (2017). Science and scepticism: Drug information, young men and counterpublic health. *Health, 21*(6), 595–615.

Fietz, H., Guedes de Mello, A., & Fonseca, C. (2020). Intimate connections and singular embodiments: disability in times of the Covid-19 pandemic. *Somatosphere*, (19 August 2020). Retrieved from http://somatosphere.net/2020/intimate-connections-singular-embodiments.html/.

Fitzgerald, D. (2020). Stay the fuck at home. *Somatosphere,* (Dispatches from the pandemic) (13 April). Retrieved from http://somatosphere.net/2020/stay-the-fuck-at-home.html/.

Ford, G. (2020). Friends are just as important as intimate partners. Allow singles to have a visitor. *Change.org petition*. Retrieved from https://www.change.org/p/victorian-premier-daniel-andrews-allow-people-living-alone-through-the-pandemic-to-form-a-bubble.

Fraser, N. (1990). Rethinking the public sphere: A contribution to the critique of actually existing democracy. *Social Text*, *25/26*, 56–80. doi:10.2307/466240

Gearin, M. (2020). Uncertainty looms for homeless Victorians in hotel accommodation during coronavirus crisis. *ABC News* (17 July). Retrieved from https://www.abc.net.au/news/2020-07-17/coronavirus-uncertainty-for-homeless-victorians-put-up-in-hotels/12464818.

Goggin, G., & Ellis, K. (2020). Disability, communication, and life itself in the COVID-19 pandemic. *Health Sociology Review*, *29*(2), 168–176. doi:10.1080/14461242.2020.1784020

HRW. (2020). Australia: Harsh police response during Covid-19. Victoria's parliament shouldn't broaden police powers. *HRW News*, (24 September). Retrieved from https://www.hrw.org/news/2020/09/24/australia-harsh-police-response-during-covid-19.

Kay, J. B. (2020). "Stay the fuck at home!": Feminism, family and the private home in a time of coronavirus. *Feminist Media Studies*, *20*(6), 883–888. doi:10.1080/14680777.2020.1765293

Lewis, S. (2020). What does the pandemic reveal about the private nuclear household? *Bullybloggers* (1 April). https://bullybloggers.wordpress.com/2020/04/01/the-virus-vs-the-home-what-does-the-pandemic-reveal-about-the-private-nuclear-household-by-sophie-lewis-for-bunkerbloggers-originally-published-on-patreon-reblogged-by-permission-of-the-author/.

Long, N. (2020). New Zealand did 'support bubbles' first. Here's what England can learn from them. *The Guardian*, (12 June). Retrieved from https://www.theguardian.com/commentisfree/2020/jun/12/new-zealand-support-bubbles-england.

McKenzie, L. (2020). Shutting down sex: COVID-19, sex and the transformation of singledom. *Anthropology in Action*, *27*(3), 9–13. doi:10.3167/aia.2020.270302

Mitchell, N. (2020). The Chief Health Officer answers dozens of your COVID-19 questions. 3AW radio interview (8 September). Retrieved from https://www.3aw.com.au/the-chief-health-officer-answers-dozens-of-your-covid-19-questions.

North Western Melbourne Primary Health Network. (2020). Stay safe, stay home. https://nwmphn.org.au/health-systems-capacity-building/covid-19/staysafe/.

Om, J. (2020). Coronavirus hard lockdown of Melbourne public housing towers left residents feeling like 'criminals', inquiry hears. *ABC News* (25 August). Retrieved from https://www.abc.net.au/news/2020-08-25/coronavirus-melbourne-public-housing-tower-shutdown-inquiry/12589372.

Race, K. (2009). *Pleasure consuming medicine: The queer politics of drugs*. Durham: Duke University Press.

Race, K. (2010). Queering HIV Prevention: An Interview with Kane Race. (12 July). Retrieved from http://www.trevorhoppe.com/blog/archives/2010/07/queering_hiv_pr.html.

Rahman, S. Y. (2020). 'Social distancing' during COVID-19: The metaphors and politics of pandemic response in India. *Health Sociology Review*, *29*(2), 131–139. doi:10.1080/14461242.2020.1790404

Rasmussen, M. L., & Leahy, D. (2018). Young people, publics and counterpublics in school-based education on gender and sexuality: An Australian story. In S. Talburt (Ed.), *Youth sexualities: Public feelings and contemporary cultural politics* (pp. 61–81). Santa Barbara: Praeger.

Roseneil, S. (2020). It's time to end the tyranny of coupledom. *The Guardian*, (14 November 2020). Retrieved from https://www.theguardian.com/commentisfree/2020/nov/14/coupledom-couple-norm-social-change.

Rubin, G. (1984). Thinking sex: Notes for a radical theory of the politics of sexuality. In C. S. Vance (Ed.), *Pleasure and danger: Exploring female sexuality* (pp. 143–178). Boston and London: Routledge and Kegan Paul.

Schlosser, A., & Harris, S. (2020). Care during COVID-19: Drug use, harm reduction, and intimacy during a global pandemic. *International Journal of Drug Policy*, *83*, 102896. doi:10.1016/j.drugpo.2020.102896

Taylor, J. (2020). 'It gets into your bones': the unique loneliness of coronavirus lockdown when you live alone. *The Guardian Australia*, (3 September). Retrieved from https://www.

theguardian.com/australia-news/2020/sep/03/it-gets-into-your-bones-the-unique-loneliness-of-coronavirus-lockdown-when-you-live-alone.

THH. (2020). Sex, Intimacy and Coronavirus Info Sheet. Retrieved from https://thorneharbour.org/covid19/sexcovid19/.

Thorneycroft, R., & Nicholas, L. (2021). Queer and crip temporalities during COVID-19: Sexual practices, risk and responsibility. In D. Lupton, & K. Willis (Eds.), *The COVID-19 crisis: Social perspectives* (pp. 103–114). London/NewYork: Routledge.

Ticktin, M. (2020). Building a Feminist Commons in the Time of COVID-19. *Signs: Feminists theorise COVID-19*. http://signsjournal.org/covid/ticktin/.

Visontay, E. (2020). What is the single social bubble in Victoria's roadmap out of Covid restrictions? *The Guardian Australia*, (9 September). Retrieved from https://www.theguardian.com/australia-news/2020/sep/09/what-is-the-single-social-bubble-in-victorias-roadmap-out-of-covid-restrictions.

Warner, M. (1999). *The trouble with normal: Sex, politics and the ethics of queer life*. Cambridge, MA: Harvard University Press.

Warner, M. (2002). Publics and counterpublics (abbreviated version). *Quarterly Journal of Speech*, *88*(4), 413–425. doi:10.1215/08992363-14-1-49

Weedon, A. (2020). Melbourne's public housing coronavirus lockdown tells a story of two cities. *ABC News*, (9 July). Retrieved from https://www.abc.net.au/news/2020-07-09/flemington-north-melbourne-public-housing-lockdown-two-cities/12431898.

Weston, K. (1997). *Families we choose: Gays, lesbians, kinship*. New York: Columbia University Press.

Domestic violence, coercive control and mental health in a pandemic: disenthralling the ecology of the domestic

Toni McCallum and Judy Rose

ABSTRACT

Domestic and family violence is a social and public health issue typically positioned in policy frameworks as a consequence of gendered social and economic structures. In this paper, we deploy an approach that draws on Hörl's neo-ecological thinking to propose that the home, as a site of domestic violence, can be usefully framed as an ecology of the domestic, a posthumanist hybrid matrix of bodies, spaces and objects in which various practices enact the smooth running of the domestic together with practices of domestic and family violence, including coercive control. Our interest is in coercive control and in the impact that the COVID-19 pandemic had on practices which enact this aspect of domestic violence. Our exploration of the practices that enact coercive control draws on the work of Law and others. We examine how practices, which are not compatible, or that do not cohere, are able to coexist in a domestic ecology and what occurs when there is a disruption as occurred with the pandemic.

Prologue

Becoming

Miranda looks around at the other mothers in the room, laughing, talking, relaxed. They hold confident and easy in their own bodies as they sip wine. Carefree like air. She isn't drinking as she has promised him she will pick up their youngest from soccer practice, do a shop and have dinner cooked before he gets home. He always has a sharp edge to him if dinner isn't ready and the kitchen is messy when he walks in the door.

A woman is standing in front of her. Talking about Miranda's new job, saying how amazing it is she can even do this with three kids and how proud and supportive her husband must have been about her getting the qualification and now working in the field. Miranda smiles and swallows hard, here we go again … … she struggles to say anything to this nice, well-dressed, woman, settling on the middle ground, 'Yeah, I love my work. It gives me a lot of satisfaction and it is a break from the kids'. Which is a lie. She never needs a break from her strong, sparky daughters. They are the reason she gets up in the morning. It is in her work that she feels competent, intelligent and valued. Nobody calls her stupid, fat, useless and a gold digger at work.

> Miranda isn't exactly sure how she went from being a confident feminist thirty something, a regular marcher on 'Reclaim the Night' rallies, to this. How she went from believing that anything was possible, that she was almost invincible, to this anxious shadow self, always trying to take up less space, always talking herself down and drawing in. Always feeling scattered in her head. Like her brain is wrapped in cloud. Constantly trying to second guess his mood. Not to upset him.
>
> But she knows it might have something to do with her relative inexperience with men. She had not had many relationships before she met him. He was tall and handsome. A highly trained professional, with a stable income. Miranda never understood why he chose her. She was so ordinary. It was like a fairytale. After she got pregnant so quickly, they moved away to Tasmania for his work, far away from her family and friends. And it was small things at first – loving how slim she got through all those years of breastfeeding and hassling her all the time when she was no longer a size 10 Barbie doll. Cutting short her phone calls to friends. Demanding sex on the first day she was back from hospital with their firstborn. Not letting her go to her friend's funeral with their first baby because it would 'disrupt the domestic routine'. Yelling at her when she visited her sister in Sydney with two toddlers, accusing her of 'abandoning the family and running away'.
>
> He was always so nice when Miranda's mother visited. In the exhausted fug of early motherhood Miranda just focused on surviving. Getting through the day. It wasn't until the kids were older that she knew something might be wrong. Seeing friends with loving, caring male partners threading small acts of kindness and gentleness through their relationships. Now she just berates herself for her lack of courage to leave. 'Just leave him for God's sake' her friend tells her. It's not that easy Miranda feels like yelling back 'I don't trust him with the kids if I'm not around'.

Miranda is a composite character created from the authors' own lived experiences and conversations with women who have experienced or worked with women exposed to coercive control as part of domestic and family violence. Miranda is modelled on Youdell's (2011) creation of a fictional composite of a disengaged schoolboy she calls 'Tommy'.

Introduction

Domestic violence is a social and public health issue that primarily (though not exclusively) affects women in intimate relationships with men (Meyer & Frost, 2019; Tomlinson, 2019). In Australia, one woman per week is killed by a man who is a current or former intimate partner (Hill, 2019, p. 7). Although more typically referred to as intimate partner violence (IPV) in North America, the more widely used and commonly accepted terms in Australia are domestic violence (Tomlinson, 2019) or domestic and family violence (Meyer & Frost, 2019; Rathus, 2013). We use these two terms interchangeably in this paper as usage has grown out of the social, policy and legal contexts across jurisdictional contexts in Australia, dating back to the 1980s (Rathus, 2013). Furthermore, the term domestic and family violence is argued to be wider in scope than IPV, but inclusive of that concept (Rathus, 2013).

As a gendered phenomenon, domestic violence is rooted in structural, social and economic inequalities that are 'gendered at the levels of social structure and interaction' (Anderson, 2010, p. 733; Dragiewicz, 2009; Elizabeth, 2015). Yet, in the tools used to assess risk for women subject to family and domestic violence, specifically coercive control, there can be a failure to recognise gender in its conceptual framing, 'thus rendering the gendered nature of risk hidden from view' (Barlow & Walklate, 2021, p. 3). The women (and fewer men) who experience domestic violence can be exposed to physical and psychological forms of abuse; the latter is conceptualised as coercive control (Stark, 2007).

Coercive control is an insidious aspect of domestic violence that can include practices of humiliation, intimidation, isolation, gaslighting (manipulating a person so that they question their actions, perceptions and abilities) as well as destroying objects and pets (Crossman, Hardesty, & Raffaelli, 2016; Fitzgerald, Barrett, Stevenson & Cheung, 2019). Yet, coercive control is often more difficult to identify compared with other forms of domestic violence, with the merits of criminalising it across all of Australia still being debated. For instance, the authors have contributed a response to the Queensland Women's Safety and Justice Taskforce (Department of Justice and Attorney-General, July 2021) call for submissions to address whether to make coercive control a standalone offence under the Queensland Domestic and Family Violence Protection Act 2012 (Rathus, Rose, Tsantefski & McCallum, 2021). By contrast, coercive control is included in the Serious Crime Act 2015 in the UK and the Domestic Abuse (Scotland) Act 2018 (Graca, 2017).

Coercive control is recognised as including psychological, financial and technology-enabled abuses that damage an individual's sense of wellbeing, self-esteem, self-confidence and faith in one's own judgement (Dragiewicz et al., 2018; Postmus, Plummer, McMahon, Murshid, & Sung Kim, 2011; Stark, 2007). Coercive control can comprise any or all of psychological, emotional, sexual and financial abuse (Stark & Hester, 2019). Financial control refers to interference with access, use and maintenance of economic resources such as money (Postmus et al., 2011). Technology-facilitated control involves behaviours such as using electronic devices and GPS applications to track and monitor a person's movement and/or interference with personal communications including via email, telephone calls, texting, and social media (Dragiewicz et al., 2018). It may also include the practice of 'doxing' which refers to unauthorised distribution of images or private information for the purposes of control, manipulation, humiliation and harm (Dragiewicz et al., 2019). Other manifestations of coercive control include the manipulation of women's relationships with children (and pets), undermining of mothering practices (Hardesty, Khaw, Ridgway, Weber, & Miles, 2013; Maher, Fitz-Gibbon, Meyer, Roberts, & Pfitzner, 2020) and restrictions on socialising, spending, personal grooming or other aspects of everyday living (Stark & Hester, 2019).

The mental health effects of coercive control are evidenced in increased rates of fear, stress, anxiety and depression amongst those who have experienced this form of abuse (Brauer, Tittle, & Antonaccio, 2019; McMahon & McGorrery, 2016). Degraded mental health may be related to restricted access to friends, family and finances along with tightening control over practices in daily life (Anderson, 2010). Such micro-regulation of daily practices often occurs within the private sphere of the home (Morison & Macleod, 2014; Rose, 2017; Rose, Brady, Yerkes, & Coles, 2015).

Some scholars argue that conditions enabling coercive control, exist within social, cultural, gendered and normative practices of romantic love, marriage and motherhood (Aisyah & Parker, 2014; Barlow & Walklate, 2021; Maher et al., 2020; McCallum,

2018). The home has consistently been found by international bodies and national researchers to be the most dangerous place for women and children (UN Women, 2020; Hill, 2019, p. 7). Maher et al. (2020) reveal the important intersections between home, family and domestic violence proffering that, 'women's roles in the family, in the building, maintenance and performance of family are consistently entangled in their experiences of family violence' (p. 13). Furthermore, socially constructed ideologies of the 'good mother' are used in abusive relationships as weapons against women to break their bonds with children (or pets) and to question their abilities as carers (Maher et al., 2020; Newberry, 2017). For example, ongoing patterns of coercive control were retrospectively exposed in the high-profile Hannah Clark case.[1]

However, despite its pervasiveness (some would say ubiquity), coercive control remains a less reported and under-researched aspect of domestic violence (Walklate & Fitz-Gibbon, 2019). A practical problem is that women's experiences of coercive control and the telling of their stories in their own words are missing from the academic literature. A previous report, *Not Now, Not Ever* (2015), chaired by Australia's then Governor General Quentin Bryce, examined domestic and family violence in Queensland and recommended that, 'stories can dramatically shift attitudes … they immerse and transport us … that act of telling assuages fear and begins healing' (Bryce, 2015, p. 81). Other research on coercive control is similarly moving towards a 'focus on the cumulative effect of the minutiae of everyday behaviours, some visible, some not, the total effect of which are abusively controlling' (Barlow & Walklate, 2021, p. 6). Telling their own stories in their own voices has been a vital part of feminist approaches. For example, Julia Kristeva's graphic, muscular, first-person poem about her own birth experience, in *Stabat Mater* (1985), is woven through her investigation of the cult of the Virgin Mary and the maternal.

Coercive control in the time of COVID-19

How did the experience of coercive control and domestic violence change for Australian women when COVID-19 was announced as a health pandemic by the World Health Organisation on 11 March 2020? An Australian research survey of 15,000 Australian women found that the rates of domestic violence had markedly increased following the outbreak of COVID-19, as had first time reports by women. In addition, 47% of women reported coercive controlling behaviours to be more frequent and severe than prior to the pandemic (Boxall, Morgan, & Brown, 2020, p. 12). Furthermore, survey results reported that women's concerns about safety were a significant barrier to them seeking outside help (Boxall et al., 2020).

Other survey research conducted with domestic violence practitioners found that while incidences of coercive control increased during the health pandemic period, this form of abuse simultaneously became less visible to the public view and more difficult for women to report to authorities (Pfitzner, Fitz-Gibbon, & True, 2020). This research found that some abusive men used COVID-19 to increase control and monitoring of women's movements and coerce them into forced cohabitation and/or breaches of social distancing (Pfitzner et al., 2020, pp. 11–12). Research further indicates that with the upsurge of pets taken in during the COVID-19 lockdown, vets were alerted to look out for increased cases of animal abuse, particularly cases where a pet becomes an object to enact control or cruelty (Boyden, Betton, Sneddon, Elliott, & Martin, 2020; Hardesty et al., 2013).

During COVID-19, domestic violence became described as a 'shadow pandemic', both globally and in Australia, as risks of abuse increased for women under the changed conditions of social isolation and forced confinement were exacerbated by financial stress, job insecurity and loss of sense of control (Fitz-Gibbon & Meyer, 2020; UN Women, 2020). Although practices of domestic violence and coercive control are situated in structural and gender inequalities that existed prior to COVID-19 (Dragiewicz, 2009), it was evident risks and harms associated with such abuses were amplified by the pandemic (Boxall et al., 2020; Pfitzner et al., 2020).

The evidence from survey research in Australia conducted during the pandemic points to COVID-19 producing new opportunities for the enactment of coercive control as well as increased incidences and risks. Given this, it is important to ask, what went on, for women like Miranda, during the global health pandemic? How did they manage in coercively controlling relationships and what were the mental health implications? In this paper, we conceptualise mental health as being co-produced in mutual relationships between people and their things, objects and environments (Cohn & Lynch, 2017). As Becker (2014) suggests, in any account of a system (in our case a home) literally everything that is there (human and non-human) is doing something (p. 3).

Miranda as method

Due to the constraints of COVID-19, we found, similar to other academics researching vulnerable families during a pandemic, it was not safe or possible to conduct formal, semi-structured, face-to-face interviews (Faircloth, Iqbal, & Twamley, 2021). This led us to explore an alternative method of using relatively unstructured interviews during the pandemic to provide us with authentic voices based on current and retrospective accounts of lived experience (Harley & Willis, 2020). Our interviewing approach used an evolving set of questions delivered more like a 'friendly conversation' (Knox & Burkard, 2009, p. 2). For example, 'I thought I'd get you to give me a bit of a narrative of the journey, before and after the whole COVID-19 flurry, and how that experience was for you?' The questions with practitioners were slightly more structured, asking questions such as 'Have you seen a difference in Domestic Violence cases you and your team have had to deal with since COVID-19?'.

Miranda then is based on an amalgamation of five women's stories, three of whom had experienced coercive control and two who worked as practitioners in the domestic and family violence sectors. All women we spoke with were white, middle-class, living in a metropolitan centre and aged between 40 and 60 years. This demographic similarity was not a deliberate strategy but indicative of the informal networks we worked through to contact women during the pandemic. Our phone and online (audio-only) interviews and conversations took place during the early stages of the COVID-19 pandemic between February and April 2020. Risks to the participants' safety were mitigated by interviews being held (without video), no partners or children present, and in a place of safety chosen by the women.

After completing the interviews, we looked to Youdell's (2011) fictional composite model of a schoolboy named 'Tommy', drawn from the common threads of a number of case studies, to create our own composite character we named 'Miranda' – a woman currently experiencing coercive control. This fictional composite approach is an effective and viscerally rich method adopted by scholars to foreground lived experience (Youdell, 2011). Miranda represents an embodied distillation of the shared lived experiences of our interview participants and allows the reader to understand the experience of coercive control from Miranda's point of view. Fostering a deeper understanding of the lived experience of coercive control and women's responses to it is an emerging theme in family and domestic violence (Walklate, Maher, McCulloch, Fitz-Gibbon, & Beavis, 2019). Moreover, through our account of Miranda we hope to illustrate that coercive control should *not* be recognised as a phenomenon that happens to 'other women', but as a set of practices that commonly take place among 'us'. The composite also allows an exploration of the interdependent web of social and material relationships with non-human entities including animals, spaces and technologies. Most importantly the composite method protects the women we spoke to by formulating a collective synthesis of the lived experience of coercive control, rather than relying on individual accounts.

What follows then is based upon our desire to provide an *holistic* account of Miranda to highlight the complexity of her circumstances that enact coercive control. To that end we turned to two sources of posthumanist thinking (Hörl, 2017, 2018; Law et al., 2014), both part of the fabric of posthumanist thought, to provide a framing of our research that accommodates the interactions of various humans and non-humans in Miranda's world.

While Law and Hörl are from two different strands in posthumanist thinking – material semiotics and neo-ecological thinking – together they gave us useful conceptual foundations with which to explore coercive control. These intellectual resources have been acknowledged as significant contributions to the posthumanist theorising of public health (Friese & Nuyts, 2017; Rock, Degeling, & Blue, 2014).

An ecology of the domestic

Influenced by the work of Hörl (2017, 2018) and Lupton (2019), we found that framing Miranda's experiences ecologically allowed us to bring to light some of the prominent, and for Miranda, risky inter-dependencies that characterised her life. We draw on Hörl's use of the notion of 'ecology' in which he argues:

> There seems to be hardly any area that cannot be considered the object of an ecology and thus open to an ecological reformulation (2017, p. 1)

Thus, thinking of the home as ecology (Hörl, 2017) draws attention to the hybridity of Miranda's world. We found a useful illustration in Hollingshead's (2020) account of the work of Mary Treat, an amateur naturalist working in the late nineteenth century of the United States. His account of Treat's work as a home-bound amateur scientist draws attention to the different practices and the various logics at play in the Treat household: logics and practices of knowledge production, social reproduction, domestic science, health and sanitation and early feminism. Hollingshead posits the home as a hybrid space of 'interlocking epistemologies' (p. 181), a *domestic ecology* (2020, pp. 181–182):

that positions the modern home as itself an ecological space – both constituted and traversed by the interactions between various human and nonhuman actants

Hollingshead depicts the ways in which Treat is able to develop practices in the home that allow her to subvert and exploit the then-dominant logics of the woman as maintainer of the home: cook, cleaner and good wife, so that she can conduct experiments, write papers and participate in scientific discourses of the time. What is of interest to us is Treat's management of logics and practices which are at odds with one another. They don't belong together. They don't fit. They are not consistent. Her kitchen is both a cooking space and her laboratory. Alongside her kitchen utensils and recipes are microscopes, insects in various stages of development and her naturalist notebooks. To the outsider, her home is not the tidy space of a well-ordered domestic environment, it is a mess. It is here we found that the work of Law et al. (2014) who examined the way in which practices that do not cohere are able to coexist, to be valuable.

Syncretism in the ecology of the domestic

Law et al. (2014) argue that all practices are syncretic, that is they are a combination of practices which operate under different, *incompatible* logics. Drawing on case studies, the authors map styles or modes in which noncoherent practices can coexist, labelling them: denial, domestication, separation, care, conflict and collapse. Law et al. (2014) offered a useful mapping for us but as we began to trace Miranda's experiences before and during the pandemic it was clear that a particular mode of syncretism, that of *separation*, was most relevant.

To illustrate, we draw attention to various attempts to manage the current pandemic. This demonstrates the bringing together of logics and their associated practices which don't easily mesh, i.e. that are syncretic. In attempts to limit and control the spread of a virus that is highly infectious and mutating regularly, health authorities have promoted practices that require significant social and economic imposts on individuals, families, organisations and businesses. The logic of prevention conveys a sense of control and reassurance communicated by the daily publication of new cases and deaths in countries that have managed to establish manageable levels of infection. While the triumph of producing vaccines in such a short time adds to the belief that the vaccine can be dealt with, in laboratories and hospitals the virus continues to be less than co-operative (Sabino et al., 2021). Improvisation, speculation and experiment run side by side as health workers struggle to help those made ill. In Law and others' terms, the noncoherence operates by masking or denying the messy and less reassuring practices of improvisation and experiment required to help people who have fallen seriously ill.

Improvisation and experiment mark the broader engagement of humans with the virus. In the home, the community and Miranda's world, new ways of doing things are deployed to counteract a virus that is yet to be domesticated. The virus runs wild. Each new variant generates new disturbances to the domestic. Each response attempts a smoothing (Halberstam, 2012). Each smoothing faces a new disturbance.

Miranda's experiences before and during the pandemic detail a posthumanistic matrix of bodies, spaces, time, pets, money and technologies that oscillates between the domestic and the wild. We describe her attempts to maintain a mode of syncretism, keeping *separate* the logics of running a smooth-running household with the logics of living with coercive control in order to achieve an appearance of domestic harmony for her children, acquaintances and extended family.

In the account that follows, we examine Miranda's domestic ecology in terms of money, space, time, technology and pets. We chose these five specific organising themes as they are foregrounded in the literature on coercive control and in the interviews (i.e. technology, Dragiewicz et al., 2018; pets, Hardesty et al., 2013; money, Postmus et al., 2011). Rock et al. (2014) also identify human relationships with the material elements 'animals, space and technology' as significant in their argument on the value of posthumanist thinking within the public health context (p. 337). In this paper, each material element we focus on in our analysis (money, space, time, technology and pets) draws attention to particular aspects of coercive control experienced by Miranda.

Just as Hollingshead's Treat is able to manage the logics and practices which are at odds with one another to be an amateur scientist *and* a good wife, Miranda, is able to adjust and adapt her practices that keep the logics of the domestic apart from the logics of coercive control.

Money

Before the pandemic

Miranda is at the supermarket check-out after having done the weekly family shop. When the check-out operator tells her the amount due, she hands him her debit card. 'Can I get $20 cash as well please.' When Miranda gets home, she hides the money in her knicker draw, in a small, bright yellow make-up purse already generously budding 10- and 20-dollar bills. Miranda saves the money so she can spend it later without having to justify or explain what she spends it on.

Money management in the home is firmly under her husband's control and oversight. Miranda has developed a way to keep the practices of a smoothly running home and the importance of discretionary spending money apart from those associated with the practices of the coercive control of money.

> Practices are noncoherent only if they are put together. If they live separate lives and never meet, then the issue of coherence or its absence never arises. We might want to say that there is a *potential* for syncretism lurking in the wings, but the potential does not get realized until, in some location or other, different practices are put together and noncoherence becomes an issue (Law et al., 2014, p. 180).

Accounting for what money has been spent on is one of the practices associated with coercive control. Even though Miranda does earn income from her part-time work, it contributes to the formal household economy. The difficulty of establishing and keeping a secret separate bank account leads Miranda to adopt the skimming practice, a modest cash economy beyond her husband's gaze. She uses the money to purchase things for herself and her children that would not be approved, deemed frivolous or unnecessary. They are items which Miranda sees as important to keeping herself and her children happy. Consumable items are the main use for this money. Items that suddenly appear in the home and for which there is no paper trail draw attention that she does not want. Even so, she occasionally still attempts purchases from the household budget prepared to put up with comments and queries like 'why did you spend all that money on that?' and, 'it's not like you earn very much of it yourself'.

Money

During the pandemic

Miranda looks in the top draw of the dresser in Freya and Kathryns' shared bedroom. She takes a new crisp $5 from the bejewelled, pink Trolls wallet. Later when she goes out, Miranda will buy a takeaway coffee. The children are not be able to spend money during COVID anyway, so she is just shifting money around their small financial ecosystem. She will pay them back when she can start skimming money again.

In the early stages of the pandemic, many supermarkets stopped the handling of money due to the uncertainty about how long the virus could stay alive on the surface of coins, paper or plastic, effectively blocking Miranda's practice of skimming. As her skimmed money becomes depleted, she adopts a workaround that maintains the separation of household spending from her discretionary spending. It's a practice that could not last for long given the modest sums in her children's wallets but it was sufficient to allow Miranda to maintain a level of discretionary spending and autonomy. In time, the supermarkets eased their restrictions on the handling of money and she was able to return to skimming. Adjustments like this are made to keep her spending practices invisible. Her circumstances allowed the maintenance of *separation.*

Space

Before the pandemic

Miranda sits at the scarred and dented wooden table and sips her green tea. The dining room is light and spacious. The opening MacBook sings the start of her work day. She can hear the dishwasher swish into its cycle. She checks to see if there are any text messages from her husband. Miranda opens her first email …

Miranda is watching Kathryn paint her Brolga model, awkwardly tipped to one side on uneven legs of paper towel cardboard cylinders. Her small face set in concentration. Miranda looks at her watch and knows she will not finish by 5pm. 'Come on hon, that looks great as it is I reckon'. Miranda must start dinner by 5 to have it on the table by 6 when he walks in. If it is not ready, he will be angry.

In use of space Miranda employs separation as the way to manage two logics, which if allowed to come together, could develop into more overt forms of domestic violence. When her husband is away at work and the children at school, it allows Miranda space to attend to various tasks, prioritised by her, and not so closely controlled by her husband. These spaces come back together at the end of the day, homework, preparing a meal and being the 'good' wife. This use of space is a delicate balancing act, one that was severely disrupted when COVID-19 arrived.

Space

During the pandemic

Miranda wakes. It is early. He is already up and working at the kitchen table doing his personal writing. Before he starts work in their bedroom where he has set up his office. He has three computer screens, a new lamp and a new office chair. Miranda goes into the kitchen to make her cup of tea. She starts rinsing the teapot and running the water. He looks up, annoyed. 'Do you have to use so much water? Why are you always so loud?' Miranda takes her teapot into the bathroom and rinses it there.

Miranda sits in the children's bunk room to work, now that her husband has set up his office space in their bedroom. Even though it is small and messy she likes the smell of sleeping children that lingers. Her daughters' homework table is small but just fits her laptop. When Miranda has her meetings sometimes the girls forget, and the dog comes into the room.

Miranda feels like these are comforting waves of the domestic nudging in and she learns to work with their rhythm.

The pandemic collapses the previous separation of the three spaces – his work, the children's school and her domestic work space. Miranda engineers a reconfigured separation and learns by trial and error how to manage any overlaps like filling a kettle in the kitchen when he is working there. She now fills the kettle in the bathroom. It's not perfect but it works.

Time

Before the pandemic

Miranda pulls on her sneakers and heads out the door for a walk. She meets her friend Helen at the corner and they chat about life and their controlling husbands. They are 3AM buddies, the first person either one calls, when things go pear-shaped.

Managing time is as important as managing the other aspects of a domestic ecology in which coercive control is in play. Building relationships and connecting with other women like her is important for Miranda's mental health and wellbeing. So too is the time she is able to commit to her part-time work which she enjoys. How she spends her time, like the money she obtains, is kept separate from time with her children and time when he is in the home. Maintaining those boundaries is not always easy.

Time

During the pandemic

He has heated the dinner Miranda prepared earlier. Her Zoom meeting with her boss is running overtime. She looks at her watch and starts to feel panicky, thinking 'can you just talk faster!' At 6.30pm he comes into the bunkroom where she's working. He says loudly 'that's enough now ... wrap it up ... dinner's on the table'
Miranda no longer feels hungry.

The pandemic has significantly diminished the discretionary time Miranda had. There are still times when she can keep things separate but there are times when the two logics clash. The interdependence of time and space means developing new practices in which she can keep separate the two logics.

Technology

Before the pandemic

Miranda switches on her laptop and logs in to the online counselling session. This is a service provided by her workplace that she confirms via a password protected work email address, not text, as she knows he checks her text messages on her phone most nights. The psychologist says 'Hello Miranda. Lovely to see you again. How have you been?' Miranda feels a wave of relief wash over her.
Later that evening Miranda comes into the kitchen and he is looking at her phone. 'What are you doing love?' Just putting 'find my phone' on your i-phone so when you lose it will be easy to find. I thought I would do it for you because you're not that technical'.

Miranda's phone and laptop are important means of maintaining connections to work and friends, but they also can be used to monitor and stalk. Miranda is not that technically minded but is aware that her texts can be easily viewed by her husband. She has no way to judge how technically adept her husband is and what other surveillance practices he has put in place. She develops practices which separate communications based upon how sensitive they may appear. Sensitive communications take place by voice and video calls at times and in spaces which are safe and away from him.

Technology

During the pandemic

It is dark and strangely quiet in the streets of their suburb as Miranda drives around. She told him she was popping out for milk from Coles before it closed. He replied 'I didn't think we needed milk. Don't forget to take your phone!'. Miranda slips the phone under papers near the front door before she leaves. She rolls down the window of the car and the air is almost sweet. Only raucous cockatoos trouble the still surface of the night …

Miranda can't call her girlfriends when he is around. She walks out to the edges of the garden to talk with neighbours. Away from his earshot, these talks are about plants, compost and COVID.

Miranda's use of her communication devices is affected by her knowledge of his surveilling practices, reading her texts and tracking her phone. Her workarounds are strictly low-tech. Her mode of syncretism remains. She is unsure how the various location tracking apps on the devices she and her husband use might be monitoring her movements. The new constraints on her time and space amplify her anxiety about the use of the various technologies she uses to communicate with others. The technology has reshaped her domestic ecology in ways that she only partially understands.

Pets

Before the pandemic

They can only have one pet in their small rented house. Although the girls want a kitten too, Miranda worries a cat could cause tension in her relationship. He barely tolerates the dog, Stan. It spends most of his time outside the house.

Pets are a common element in many households, an integral part of the domestic ecology. However, different species require different practices to generate the companionship they provide humans. For Miranda, having Stan in the house is problematic when he is at home. She enjoys the dog's company even when it interrupts her when she is working. She does not understand his attitude towards pets but as long as Stan spends most of his time in the back yard, out of sight and mind mostly, things are calm.

Pets

During the pandemic

Miranda acquires a COVID kitten, Winston, at the insistence of her girls who are isolated from their friends. Days after acquiring the kitten, she sees him behind the shed, a shovel is on the ground next to a pile of soil. Miranda feels her neck prickle as she stares down at the small body. It doesn't look like Winston as he is rigid and strangely buckled in the shallow grave, 'Oh I had to break his leg to get him in'. Miranda asks how he died. 'Oh, he must have got on the road'. Winston never goes near the road. Miranda feels sick and walks away. She wonders what she will tell the girls.

During the pandemic, the acquisition of pets surged (Morgan et al., 2020). Isolation from usual contacts was in part replaced by new animal–human relationships. Acquiring Winston seemed a logical move for Miranda even though she was wary of his reaction to a pet that spent most of its time indoors. Maintaining a separation, as she had achieved with Stan, was more difficult. The two logics collapsed. The outcome was violent.

Miranda (and women like her) in a pandemic

Our interest in the documented rise in domestic violence against women during the current pandemic prompted this research. What was going on that brought about the change in the frequency of domestic violence? It is easy to speculate about what was going on. We chose to look at coercive control, a serious form of domestic violence in itself, and often a precursor to more overt acts of violence. To do this, we created a composite character we called Miranda, loosely based on the women we interviewed, and described the practices she had in place before the pandemic and how they changed during the pandemic. Using small, poetic, intensely personal stories, we reveal how Miranda traversed the socio-material practices of coercive control.

Our descriptions of Miranda's lived experience illustrate how pandemic conditions complicated her management of controlling practices (e.g. not being able to skim money from the supermarket so easily, impeding her freedom of movement). COVID-19 further eroded Miranda's already fragile mental health and she had greater difficulty accessing her counsellor and other vital supports. Our approach has allowed a nuanced detailing of coercive controlling practices under the lockdown conditions of a pandemic. As Becker (2014) suggests 'the richest sociological possibilities [lie] in the smallest details of the stories' (p. 3). Hollingshead's analysis drew our attention to Mary Treat's management of what we called logics that did not easily cohere or not cohere at all.

We drew on the work of Law et al. (2014) to describe how the two logics evident in Miranda's domestic ecology and which were clearly noncoherent, that of the smoothly running home and that of a coercively controlling husband, were managed by Miranda. It was clear that the mode of syncretism Miranda deployed was one of keeping the two logics apart, of separation. The pandemic disrupted all of the strategies Miranda had developed to maintain separation. The perturbation of the posthumanistic matrix of bodies, spaces, time, pets, money and technologies was countered in most instances thereby avoiding a virus-induced *wilding* of her domestic ecology.

For our composite Miranda, practices that kept the two logics apart remained her mode of choice during the pandemic. For the most part, she was able to maintain the separation that allowed the performance of the home as a secure, safe and smoothly running place and manage her mental health. Miranda's preservation of self (and self-care) is evidenced in subtle practices such as deliberately leaving her mobile phone at home and in accessing secret sources of money for discretionary spending and confidential counselling at work. Similarly, other women living with coercive control 'will and do get on with their lives' (Barlow & Walklate, 2021, p. 14). For other Mirandas, the maintenance of keeping the logics separate may not have been as successful as the statistics indicate.

As is the case for all victims of coercive control, significant disruptions, like the current pandemic, will make previously successful strategies unworkable. Miranda's reinvention of her syncretic practices illustrates how difficult, dangerous and tenuous developing new practices can be.

Note

1. The 2020 case of Brisbane woman Hannah Clark (and her children) murdered by estranged husband Rowan Baxter, who incinerated his whole family, before killing himself. This case has brought the phenomenon of coercive control to the forefront because it shows how coercively controlling practices including psychological, economic and emotional abuse enacted through intimidation, digital surveillance and stalking can spiral into extreme physical violence and/or death.

Acknowledgements

The authors would like to express their deepest gratitude and thanks to their mentor Prof. Chris Bigum. His comments on our writing and theory development were invaluable.

Disclosure statement

No potential conflict of interest was reported by the author(s).

Funding

The author(s) reported there is no funding associated with the work featured in this article.

ORCID

Judy Rose http://orcid.org/0000-0001-6383-7666

References

Aisyah, S., & Parker, L. (2014). Problematic conjugations: Women's agency, marriage and domestic violence in Indonesia. *Asian Studies Review*, *38*(2), 205–223.

Anderson, K. L. (2010). Conflict, power, and violence in families. *Journal of Marriage and Family*, *72*(3), 726–742.

Barlow, C., & Walklate, S. (2021). Gender, risk assessment and coercive control: Contradictions in terms? *The British Journal of Criminology*, *61*, 887–904. doi:10.1093/bjc/azaa104

Becker, H. S. (2014). What about Mozart? What about murder?. *Revista Brasileira de Ciências Sociais*, *29*(86), 5–13.

Boxall, H., Morgan, A. & Brown, R. (2020). *The prevalence of domestic violence among women during the COVID-19 pandemic.* Statistical Bulletin no. 28. Canberra: Australian Institute of Criminology. Retrieved from https://www.aic.gov.au/publications/sb/sb28

Boyden, P., Betton, V., Sneddon, W., Elliott, M., & Martin, D. (2020). Increase in animal abuse likely during lockdown. *The Veterinary Record*, *186*(14), 457.

Brauer, J. R., Tittle, C. R., & Antonaccio, O. (2019). The costs of coercive control: Assessing behavioral and mental health correlates of erratic and oppressive coercion. *Justice Quarterly*, *36*(2), 255–286.

Cohn, S., & Lynch, R. (2017). Posthuman perspectives: Relevance for a global public health. *Critical Public Health*, *27*(3), 285–292.

Crossman, K. A., Hardesty, J. L., & Raffaelli, M. (2016). "He could scare me without laying a hand on me" Mothers' experiences of nonviolent coercive control during marriage and after separation. *Violence Against Women*, *22*(4), 454–473.

Dragiewicz, M. (2009). Why sex and gender matter in domestic violence research and advocacy. In E. Stark, & E. Buzawa (Eds.), *Violence against women in families and relationships: Vol. 3: Criminal justice and the law* (pp. 201–215). Santa Barbara, CA: Praeger.

Dragiewicz, M., Burgess, J., Matamoros-Fernández, A., Salter, M., Suzor, N. P., Woodlock, D., & Harris, B. (2018). Technology facilitated coercive control: Domestic violence and the competing roles of digital media platforms. *Feminist Media Studies, 18*(4), 609–625.

Dragiewicz, M., Harris, B., Woodlock, D., Salter, M., Easton, H., Lynch, A., Campbell, H., Leach, J. & Milne, L., (2019). *Domestic violence and communication technology: Survivor experiences of intrusion, surveillance, and identity crime*. Sydney: Australian Communications Consumer Action Network & Queensland University of Technology.

Elizabeth, V. (2015). From domestic violence to coercive control: Towards the recognition of oppressive intimacy in the family court. *New Zealand Sociology, 30*(2), 26.

Faircloth, C., Iqbal, H., & Twamley, K. (2021). *'Er, not the best time': The challenges of researching family life during a pandemic-transforming society*. Transforming Society. Bristol University Press & Policy Press. Retrieved from https://www.transformingsociety.co.uk/2021/01/13/er-not-the-best-time-the-challenges-of-researching-family-life-during-a-pandemic/

Fitzgerald, A. J., Barrett, B. J., Stevenson, R., & Cheung, C. H. (2019). Animal maltreatment in the context of intimate partner violence: A manifestation of power and control?. *Violence Against Women, 25*(15), 1806–1828.

Fitz-Gibbon, K., & Meyer, S. (2020). *Coronavirus: Fear of family violence spike as COVID-19 impact hits households*. Monash Lens. Retrieved from https://lens.monash.edu/@politics-society/2020/03/18/1379841/coronavirus-fear-of-family-violence-spikeas-covid-19-impact-hits-households

Friese, C., & Nuyts, N. (2017). Posthumanist critique and human health: How nonhumans (could) figure in public health research. *Critical Public Health, 27*(3), 303–313. doi:10.1080/09581596.2017.1294246

Graca, S. (2017). Domestic violence policy and legislation in the UK: A discussion of immigrant women's vulnerabilities. *European Journal of Current Legal Issues, 22*, 1.

Halberstam, J. (2012). *Gaga feminism: Sex, gender, and the end of normal*. Boston: Beacon Press.

Hardesty, J. L., Khaw, L., Ridgway, M. D., Weber, C., & Miles, T. (2013). Coercive control and abused women's decisions about their pets when seeking shelter. *Journal of Interpersonal Violence, 28*, 2617–2639.

Harley, K., & Willis, K. (2020). Living with motor neurone disease: An insider's sociological perspective. *Health Sociology Review, 29*, 211–225. doi:10.1080/14461242.2020.1789487

Hill, J. (2019). *See what you made me do: Power, control and domestic abuse*. Carlton, Victoria: Black Inc.

Hollingshead, D. (2020). Women, insects, modernity: American domestic ecologies in the late nineteenth century. *Feminist Modernist Studies, 3*(2), 180–204.

Hörl, E. (2017). Introduction to general ecology: The ecologization of thinking (N. F. Schott, Trans.). In E. Hörl, & J. Burton (Eds.), *General ecology: The new ecological paradigm* (pp. 1–74). London, UK: Bloomsbury Academic.

Hörl, E. (2018). General ecology. In R. Braidotti, & M. Hlavajova (Eds.), *Posthuman glossary* (pp. 172–175). London, UK: Bloomsbury Academic.

Knox, S., & Burkard, A. W. (2009). Qualitative research interviews. *Psychotherapy Research, 19*(4-5), 566–575.

Kristeva, J. (1985). Stabat mater. In T. Moi (Ed.), *The Kristeva reader: Julia Kristeva* (pp. 160–186). Oxford: Basil Blackwell.

Law, J., Afdal, G., Asdal, K., Lin, W. Y., Moser, I., & Singleton, V. (2014). Modes of syncretism: Notes on noncoherence. *Common Knowledge, 20*(1), 172–192.

Lupton, D. (2019). Toward a more-than-human analysis of digital health: Inspirations from feminist new materialism. *Qualitative Health Research, 29*(14), 1998–2009.

Maher, J., Fitz-Gibbon, K., Meyer, S., Roberts, S., & Pfitzner, N. (2020). Mothering through and in violence: Discourses of the 'good mother'. *Sociology*. doi:10.1177/0038038520967262

McCallum, T. (2018) *(M)other love: Cultural difference and gendered practices in Queensland, Australia* (Doctoral thesis). University of Newcastle, Nova dissertations and Theses Global.

McMahon, M., & McGorrery, P. (2016). Criminalising controlling and coercive behaviour: The next step in the prosecution of family violence? *Alternative Law Journal, 41*(2), 98–101.

Meyer, S., & Frost, A. (2019). *Domestic and family violence: A critical introduction to knowledge and practice*. New York: Routledge.

Morgan, L., Protopopova, A., Birkler, R. I. D., Itin-Shwartz, B., Sutton, G. A., Gamliel, A., Raz, T. (2020). Human–dog relationships during the COVID-19 pandemic: Booming dog adoption during social isolation. *Humanities and Social Sciences Communications*, *7*(1), 155. doi:10.1057/s41599-020-00649-x

Morison, T., & Macleod, C. (2014). When veiled silences speak: Reflexivity, trouble and repair as methodological tools for interpreting the unspoken discourse-based data. *Qualitative Research*, *14*, 694–711.

Newberry, M. (2017). Pets in danger: Exploring the link between domestic violence and animal abuse. *Aggression and Violent Behavior*, *34*, 273–281.

Pfitzner, N., Fitz-Gibbon, K., & True, J. (2020). *Responding to the 'Shadow Pandemic': Practitioner views on the nature of and responses to violence against women in Victoria, Australia during the COVID-19 restrictions*. doi:10.26180/5ed9d5198497c

Postmus, J. L., Plummer, S.-B., McMahon, S., Murshid, N. S., & Sung Kim, M. (2011). Understanding economic abuse in the lives of survivors. *Journal of Interpersonal Violence*. doi:10.1177/0886260511421669

Rathus, Z. (2013). Shifting language and meanings between social science and the law: Defining family violence. *University of New South Wales Law Journal*, *36*(2), 359–389.

Rathus, Z., Rose, J., Tsantefski, M., & McCallum, T. (2021). *Submission to women's safety and justice taskforce options for legislating against coercive control and the creation of a standalone domestic violence offence*. Discussion Paper 1. July, 2021. https://www.womenstaskforce.qld.gov.au

Rock, M. J., Degeling, C., & Blue, G. (2014). Toward stronger theory in critical public health: Insights from debates surrounding posthumanism. *Critical Public Health*, *24*(3), 337–348. doi:10.1080/09581596.2013.827325

Rose, J. (2017). "Never enough hours in the day": Employed mothers' perceptions of time pressure. *Australian Journal of Social Issues*, *52*(2), 116–130.

Rose, J., Brady, M., Yerkes, M. A., & Coles, L. (2015). "Sometimes they just want to cry for their mum": Couples' negotiations and rationalisations of gendered divisions in infant care. *Journal of Family Studies*, *21*(1), 38–56.

Sabino, E. C., Buss, L. F., Carvalho, M. P. S., Prete, C. A., Crispim, M. A. E., & Fraiji, N. A. (2021). Resurgence of COVID-19 in Manaus, Brazil, despite high seroprevalence. *The Lancet*, *397*, 452–455. doi:10.1016/SO140-6736(21)00183-5

Special Taskforce on Domestic and Family Violence in Queensland, & Bryce, Q. (2015). *Not now, not ever: Putting an end to domestic and family violence in Queensland*. Brisbane: Queensland Government.

Stark, E. (2007). *Coercive control: How men entrap women in personal life*. Oxford: Oxford University Press.

Stark, E. & Hester, M. (2019). Coercive control: Update and review. *Violence Against Women*, *25* (1), 81–104.

Tomlinson, J. (2019). Domestic violence is a major public health issue. *Australian Medicine*, *31* (14), 14.

UN Women. (2020). *Violence against women and girls: the shadow pandemic*. Retrieved from https://www.unwomen.org/en/news/stories/2020/4/statement-ed-phumzile-violence-against-women-during-pandemic.

Walklate, S., & Fitz-Gibbon, K. (2019). The criminalisation of coercive control: The power of law? *International Journal for Crime, Justice and Social Democracy*, *8*(4), 94.

Walklate, S., Maher, J., McCulloch, J., Fitz-Gibbon, K., & Beavis, K. (2019). Victim stories and victim policy: Is there a case for a narrative victimology? *Crime, Media, Culture*, *15*(2), 199–215.

Youdell, D. (2011). *School trouble: Identity, power and politics in education*. New York: Routledge.

Lost in translation? Beyond sex as a biological variable in animal research

Madeleine Pape

ABSTRACT

In this article, I develop a feminist posthumanist account of biomedical policymaking as a material-discursive intervention that shapes the emergence of phenomena in the scientific laboratory. The setting is United States (U.S.) biomedicine, where a recent policy of the National Institutes of Health has mandated the consideration of sex in basic and preclinical research. Called Sex as a Biological Variable (SABV), the mandate configures cell lines and animal models as the next frontier in the project of advancing gender equity in biomedical research. Given sex and gender are increasingly recognised as having complex, entangled, and dynamic effects on human health and illness, how do laboratory animals respond to their attempted enrolment in this regulatory intervention? Through a qualitative analysis of this policy domain, I show how laboratory animals reveal the context-specific character of sex, its multiplicity and elusiveness as a so-called biological variable, and the considerable work needed to shore up human ideologies of sex as a pervasive cross-species form of binary difference. I suggest that while regulatory interventions constrain patterns of mattering, they also serve as agential openings in which laboratory animals can 'kick back' and reconfigure the pursuit of knowledge, particularly as it relates to difference and health.

> Actors come in many and wonderful forms. Accounts of a 'real' world do not, then, depend on a logic of 'discovery', but on a power-charged social relation of 'conversation'. (Haraway, 1988, p. 593)

> Sex-based research can be a powerful tool for discovery. Studying both sexes can unveil biological truths, new fundamental knowledge, and new biological mechanisms. – NIH Office of Research on Women's Health (ORWH, 2014a, p. 23)

In October 2014, scientists from across North America gathered with policymakers at the United States (U.S.) National Institutes of Health (NIH) for a workshop centred on a new mandate aimed at making 'sex' foundational to the nation's biomedical enterprise. Called Sex as a Biological Variable (SABV), the policy elevates sex as a key determinant of health whose study begins at the basic and preclinical level (Clayton & Collins, 2014; NIH, 2015). In summarising the workshop's proceedings, NIH policymakers emphasised 'the importance of addressing biological sex as a variable as part of the larger NIH effort to ensure rigor and reproducibility in research,' since '[b]iological sex, being female or male, is a fundamental characteristic of biological systems' (ORWH, 2014a, pp. 2–4). Yet many questions raised during the workshop remained unanswered, including: how is 'sex' distinct from 'gender,' how does it vary, how can its mechanisms be studied in cell lines – if at all – and with what relevance to human experiences of health and illness? In short, how can biomedical researchers account for the complexity of sex and its varied, dynamic, and indeterminate presence both within and beyond the laboratory?

This article approaches the SABV mandate as an opportunity to examine the role of 'nonhuman' entities, and particularly laboratory animals, in shaping how biomedical researchers and policymakers enact accounts of embodied difference and its relationship to health.[1] A core insight from Science and Technology Studies (STS) is that the pursuit of scientific knowledge requires the enrolment of heterogeneous human and nonhuman objects (Callon, 1984; Callon & Law, 1997; Latour, 2005). As such, any attempt to sociologically explain how certain scientific research agendas come to emerge at particular moments in time ought also to account for the material objects and non-human elements upon which such agendas depend (Latour, 2000). According to Bruno Latour, 'it is always things … which, in practice, lend their "steely" quality to the hapless "society"' (Latour, 2005, p. 68). Such objects are not merely passively enrolled in projects of scientific knowledge-making: they are frequently recalcitrant, resisting the efforts of scientists to master them (Latour, 2000). By attending to how these wily entities participate (or not) in the scientific enterprise, social scientists can reveal the negotiations involved in establishing certain knowledge claims as scientific 'facts.'

A similar orientation to nonhuman agency is found within feminist science studies. Donna Haraway (1988) calls for feminists to engage their material world as 'Coyote or Trickster:' a 'witty agent and actor' that is ever eluding efforts at mastery and control (pp. 593–6). To Haraway, the task is to not only render visible these nonhuman actors but to *learn to converse*: 'to become capable, with each other in all our bumptious kinds, of *response*' (Haraway, 2016, p. 1, emphasis added). In developing this 'response-ability' (p. 2), new ways of living with and knowing the world might be realised. Extending this logic to the scientific and regulatory pursuit of sex as a biological variable, we might ask whether engaging differently with model organisms in the laboratory would generate new insights about what sex as a health determinant is presumed to be. What, too, might we learn about where and how nonhuman entities are relied upon to construct ideologies of female/male difference in humans?

As Linda Birke (2010) has observed, for all their careful attention to the problematic ways that scientists enact sex, feminist science studies scholars have less often approached laboratory animals as offering valuable insights into the contingent character of scientific claims about binary female/male difference. Perhaps for fear of affirming the biological determinism they seek to repudiate, they have at times avoided engaging with non-human animals, even though the science they critique is very often influenced by animal research (Birke, Bryld, & Lykke, 2004). I take up Birke's challenge to engage non-human entities as central to scientific claims about biological sex, looking to the policy work surrounding the SABV mandate as a unique empirical opportunity for doing so. In the process, I develop a feminist –

and posthumanist – account of biomedical policymaking as a material-discursive intervention that sociologists can study to better understand the 'entanglements of human and non-human bodies, affects, objects and cultural practices' that underpin the production of health knowledge (Fullagar, 2017, p. 248). That is, following Karen Barad (2007), policymaking can be conceptualised as a regulatory practice that necessarily engages diverse material entities *and* has material effects in the world, calling for new modes of sociological response-ability.

Drawing on a range of qualitative materials, I show how the non-human entities called upon to affirm the SABV policy in fact lend their support to key insights from feminist science studies, namely the inherently political character of scientific knowledge production, the entanglement of gender ('the social') and sex ('the biological'), and the complex non-dimorphic (and always context-specific) ways that sex can be shown to vary. I conclude by considering the implications for how biomedical researchers, policymakers, and sociologists might engage with and learn from non-human entities in the pursuit of knowledge about human health.

Policy enactments of sex as a biological variable

Implemented in 2016, the SABV policy applies to preclinical research involving vertebrate animals, though researchers using cell lines, primary cells, or tissue explants are also asked to account for sex (NIH, 2018). It positions the NIH as the first funding agency in the world to grant sex its own dedicated inclusion policy, though agencies in other contexts such as Canada and the European Union have since adopted a similar approach (Gendered Innovations, 2020). The mandate requires researchers to explain how sex will be factored into research designs and analyses, with the expectation that they include both female and male animals (or offer strong justification for not doing so) and disaggregate their data by sex (NIH, 2015). In this way, it builds on but is also distinct from earlier mandates for inclusion in US biomedicine, most notably the NIH Revitalization Act of 1993, which focused on clinical trial research and sought to remedy the perceived over-reliance on middle-aged white men (Epstein, 2007). Unlike these previous eras of policymaking, the SABV policy targets animal and cell research and specifies sex alone as a master 'biological variable' deemed universally relevant across the research spectrum.

While the SABV policy has been heralded by its proponents as a significant feat for women's health (Clayton, 2016a; SWHR, 2015), a second purpose of the mandate is to address concerns regarding the reproducibility of basic and preclinical research. In 2012, researchers revealed in *Nature* that of 53 'landmark' studies in the fields of hematology and oncology, they could only reproduce six (Begley & Ellis, 2012). By 2014, NIH leadership declared that 'the complex system for ensuring the reproducibility of biomedical research is failing and is in need of restructuring' (Collins & Tabak, 2014, p. 612). Amongst the range of factors believed to be compromising animal studies in particular, NIH policymakers identified an 'incomplete understanding of potential sex-based differences' (NIH, 2015). In short, it is believed that researchers will be better able to master animal models once the presence and effects of sex have been properly accounted for. Delivering on this promise, however, requires the cooperation of the animals around which laboratory practices are organised.

Towards regulation as material-discursive intervention

To develop a feminist approach to biomedical policymaking as a material-discursive intervention with implications for human/nonhuman (and sociological) response-ability, I combine three areas of STS and posthumanist scholarship. The first is Sarah Richardson's (2021) concept of *sex contextualism*: the notion that what sex is, and how it is operationalised by scientists, depends upon the research context and the specific research questions being pursued. Second, I draw on Barad's (2003, 2007) framework of *agential intra-action* to account for the material-discursive nature of laboratory phenomena and the role of technoscientific practices therein. Third, I approach the regulation of biomedical research as one such technoscientific practice that has material effects in the laboratory and the world (Epstein, 2007; Jasanoff, 2005). Taken together, I suggest that rule-making moments such as the SABV policy allow for the sociological examination of how regulatory practices attempt to engage nonhuman entities in the pursuit of particular institutional, political, and scientific ends.

A considerable body of feminist STS scholarship has revealed that variation across the traits popularly associated with sex does not amount to a neatly binary female/male classification (Fausto-Sterling, 2000; Karkazis, 2019). From the complex workings of testosterone in the body, to the dynamic formation of gender-linked variation in the brain, to the inconclusive role of X and Y chromosomes in determining female and male bodies, feminist scholars have shown sex to be an indeterminate, overlapping, and responsive form of embodied variation (Hyde et al., 2019; Jordan-Young, 2012; Jordan-Young & Karkazis, 2019; Richardson, 2013). Scientists must therefore engage in considerable work to override 'awkward surpluses' of unruly data and align their findings with expectations of a binary model of sex difference (Fujimura, 2006, p. 51). This is not to suggest that biological factors play no role in shaping trajectories of health and illness. Rather, feminist scholars presume from the outset that 'biology' varies in complex ways and is always already dynamically entangled with social processes (Krieger, 2003; Ritz et al., 2014; Springer, Stellman, & Jordan-Young, 2012).

Richardson's concept of sex contextualism attempts to account for the complexity of sex in the scientific laboratory (see also Eliot & Richardson, 2016). She suggests that biomedical researchers would be best served by recognising that:

> [T]he definition of sex and sex-related variables, and whether they are relevant in biological research, depends on the research context. This research context may include pragmatic interests, observational constraints, interacting or mediating environmental variables, characters of the species or strain, developmental stage of the research organism or materials, and level of biological analysis—for example, cell, tissue, organism, and community. Whether and how 'sex' is operationalized will be specific to each experimental setting ... there is no 'sex itself.' There is only sex as pragmatically constituted in an observational frame. (2021, p. 21)

This context-specific approach to sex is highly relevant to animal research, where the experimental outcomes of interest to researchers are shaped by diverse factors such as the specific species or strain, how animals are housed and handled, and other laboratory and experimental conditions (Birke, 2010; Birke et al., 2004; Fausto-Sterling, 2000; Gungor, Duchesne, & Bluhm, 2019; Terry, 2000). A classic example is the relationship between cage size and sexual response: when female rats are space-constrained, they are more likely to exhibit lordosis – the posture permitting coitus – rather than other more active sexual behaviours (Birke, 2010). Experimental design can thus reproduce the notion of the passive female and inhibit the discovery of traits that might support alternative notions of femininity/masculinity.

Where and how might the regulation of biomedical research fit within a contextual approach to sex? As various STS scholars have argued – and feminist scholars increasingly recognise – policymaking practices generate the conditions that enable the production of *certain* forms of scientific knowledge while disabling others (Epstein, 2007; Frickel et al., 2009; Jasanoff, 2005; Karkazis, 2019; Pape, 2021). A useful organising concept to account for this relationship is Barad's (2003, 2007) posthumanist notion of 'intra-action,' which calls attention to the heterogeneous elements that comprise and produce 'phenomena' in the laboratory:

> [T]he primary ontological unit [in the scientific laboratory] is not independent objects with inherent boundaries and properties but rather *phenomena* … phenomena do not merely mark the epistemological inseparability of observer and observed, or the results of measurements; rather, *phenomena are the ontological inseparability/entanglement of intra-acting 'agencies.'* (Barad, 2007, p. 139, emphasis in original).

That is, laboratory phenomena implicate not a separate observer, observed object, and measuring apparatus but rather their intra-active co-constitution. So, too, does Barad consider regulatory practices to be material-discursive interventions that form part of the 'iterative intra-activity of the world in its becoming' (2007, p. 152). In addition to their generative enabling effects, they may serve as important boundary-drawing instruments or 'agential cuts' (2007, p. 140) that impose '[m]aterial constraints and exclusions' and influence which components of phenomena are recognised as determinate and meaningful (2003, p. 815). For example, regulatory practices may shape the delineation of 'human' from 'nonhuman,' 'culture' from 'nature,' and 'science' from 'the social' (2007, p. 140).

As Simone Fullagar (2017) has argued, these are dualisms that health sociologists, too, have at times unreflexively reified. Fullagar calls on sociologists to develop an alternative ethico-onto-epistemological sensibility in which they 'critically challenge, rather than unknowingly reiterate, normative assumptions' (p. 248) about the boundaries of the human body and the 'matter' that matters to human health. I suggest that sociologists can approach the boundary-drawing efforts implicated in policymaking as a means to investigate where and how 'the world kicks back' (Barad, 2007, p. 215). That is, while such practices may constrain response-ability, they also serve as valuable conversation opportunities, in the case of the SABV policy creating what I call *agential openings* in which it becomes possible to reimagine dominant (human) notions of what sex is and how it is presumed to vary.

Data and methods

In the analysis to follow, I conceptualise biomedical policymaking as implicating a variety of human (and non-human) actors located both within and external to the NIH itself (Epstein, 2007; Hess, 2004). I focus primarily on the activities of the ORWH – established in 1990 to promote women's health research both within and beyond the NIH – and their Advisory Committee for Research on Women's Health (ACRWH), a group of invited researchers and advisors who provide input on NIH policy priorities. I rely primarily on transcripts of key meetings in which the SABV policy was discussed, policy statements produced by ORWH policymakers, biomedical researchers, and policy advisors, and peer-reviewed journal articles relied upon to justify the SABV policy as a legitimate mandate for animal research. These data were supplemented by ACRWH meeting minutes (1994–2016), responses to a 2014 NIH call for stakeholder input in the SABV policy (NIH, 2014), and media coverage of the mandate.

Across these texts, I examine how the nonhuman entities of the scientific laboratory are frequently presumed to be passive background actors, leveraged primarily to justify how and why the SABV policy ought to be implemented and with what benefit for women and the U.S. biomedical enterprise. And yet the considerable complexity of animal models – and researchers' relations to them – also rise to the surface, often in ways that reveal the limitations of the SABV policy as an intervention intended to advance health knowledge.

Modelling gender politics

A central tenet of feminist science studies is that enactments of sex in the scientific laboratory are shaped by the ideological assumptions that researchers bring to bear on their experiments, influencing which research questions are deemed worth asking, how studies are designed, and how data is interpreted and presented (Keller, 1985; Martin, 1991; Richardson, 2013). Here the science in question is already pursuing sex, as in the case of Joan Fujimura's (2006) analysis of research examining so-called sex determining genes (the 'SRY' and 'DAX-1' genes) in mice and humans. The case of the SABV policy sheds light on a different way that gender politics shape scientific research: namely, the *avoidance* of studying sex, often because of the androcentric assumption that male models offer universal insights (Epstein, 2007). Enter the posthumanist feminist politics of animal research: how to do it *well*, in ways that neither reify sex nor avoid biology altogether (Birke, 2010)?

The existence of a male bias in animal research is well documented, with some fields characterised by a ratio as high as a 5–1 in favour of male models (Zucker & Beery, 2010).[2] This pervasive androcentrism was even recognised by comedian Steven Colbert following the SABV policy announcement: the 'longstanding tradition of testing on only male animals is based on the assumption that females are simply a variation on a theme. Folks, that's science. Male is default human' (The Colbert Report, 2014).[3] The reasons are all too familiar to advocates of women's inclusion in biomedical research: 'convention', and perceptions that the estrus cycle of female mammals (and human females) makes them too variable to be worthy research subjects (Clayton & Collins, 2014).

In recent years, animal models have in fact proven instrumental to debunking the gendered myth of female variability. A 2014 study by Brian Prendergast and colleagues analysed 293 articles to determine whether free-cycling female mice (included without controlling for the stage of their estrous cycle) were more variable than males. Across a wide range of behavioural, morphological, physiological, and molecular traits, the authors found that not only did trait variability in females never significantly exceed that of males, but that females were significantly *less* variable than males for three trait categories (hormonal, metabolism-related, and morphological) (Figure 1). That is, in a reversal of the dominant assumption, male mice can be *more* hormonally variable

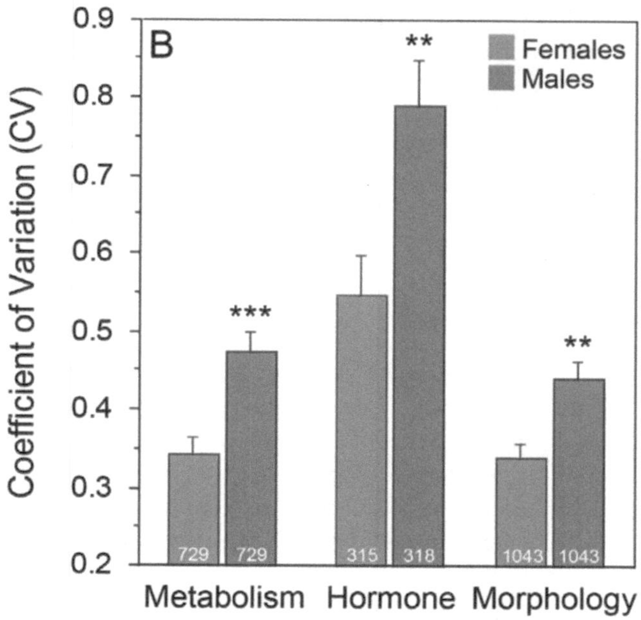

Figure 1. Lower variability in females compared to males for hormonal, metabolism-related, and morphological traits. (Prendergast, Onishi, & Zucker, 2014, p. 3).

than free-cycling females. The authors also analysed the role of housing conditions on trait variability, finding that group-housed mice (both female and male) were more hormonally variable than their single-housed peers.[4] Yet even amongst single-housed mice, females were no more variable than males, suggesting laboratory mice can be allies in feminist efforts to reveal the gendered material-discursive practices of science.

Yet policy discussions also reveal that animal models do *sometimes* reveal *something* that approximates what scientific researchers might under *certain circumstances* refer to in the shorthand as 'sex.' A consistent story shared by biomedical researchers is that, rather than setting out to pursue the workings of sex in their animal models, they were ultimately faced with no choice but to engage it. Consider the account of Louise McCollough, stroke researcher and neuroscientist, during a 2015 panel on the SABV policy (ACRWH, 2015):

> I was looking at this particular mouse strain ... which had been shown in a *Science* paper to be protected against stroke in an ischemic injury. I started to do the females and I was looking at estrogen and [the experiment] just didn't work. It drove me batty ... The next year I did hundreds and hundreds of Parp [knockout] mice ... it was after probably two and a half years I realized that it is not me. I was not flawed in doing these [experiments]. It was not the mouse. It was that there was a sex difference.

Bacteriologist Heather Cross shared a similar accidental discovery of sex-linked mechanisms after being forced to work with female mice: '[T]here was a remarkable difference which led to a whole cascade of studies looking at how females could be protected from myocardial infarction via various ionic pathways ... We would have come up with remarkably different conclusions had we not looked at both sexes.'

Thus, which animals are deemed to 'matter' is inseparable from the broader gendered context within which researchers are located (Bleier, 1984). For their part, wily laboratory animals may sometimes reveal unexpected variation, while at other times show that the assumption of variation (or its direction) was misplaced from the outset. Yet here we must tread carefully: if it is indeed 'sex' that laboratory animals are (sometimes) revealing, how can it be recognised as context-specific and contingent rather than universal and omnipresent (Richardson, 2021)?

Gendering laboratory relations

Underpinning the SABV policy is the assumption that sex is a 'biological variable:' one whose effects can be studied independently of gender and other contextual (and particularly social) factors. It is frequently defined by proponents of the SABV policy in such terms as 'based on biology—derived from sex chromosomes and corresponding gonadal structures, and declared at birth,' whereas gender is 'a psychosocial construct that encompasses how one views oneself,' 'gender identity,' or 'the societal and cultural context that assigns certain roles (gender role) and behaviours to individuals' (Brooks & Clayton, 2016, p. 15). This analytical distinction between sex and gender is deemed crucial to the success of the SABV policy, given decades of conflation of the two terms amongst both scientists and federal legislators (Epstein, 2007; Pape, 2021). It has also enabled NIH policymakers to argue that whereas gender is only relevant in the latter stages of the research spectrum, sex is relevant throughout (Figure 2).

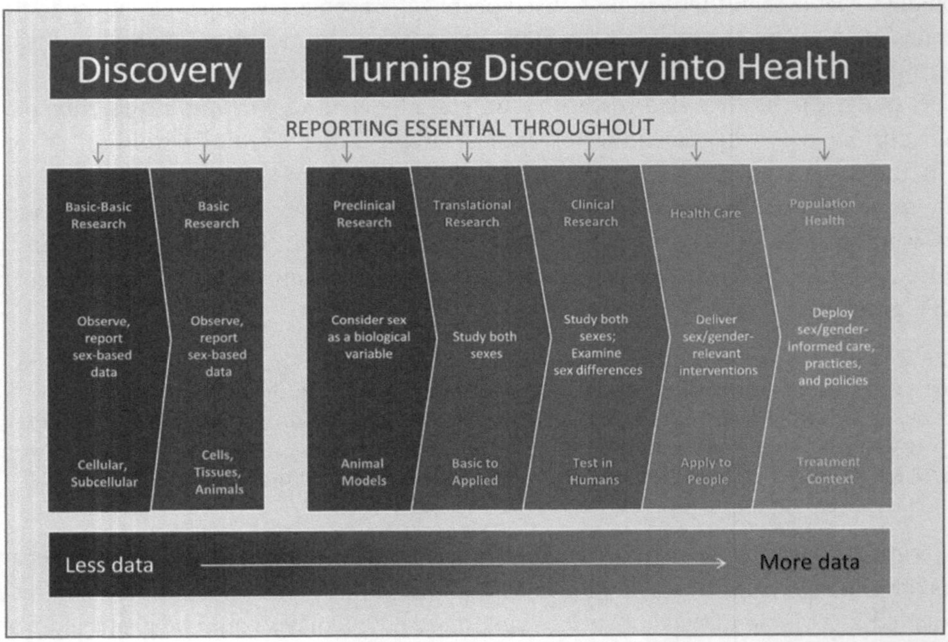

Figure 2. Total integration of sex and restricted integration of gender across the biomedical research spectrum (Clayton, 2016b, p. 520).

Animal models allegedly provide the evidence to justify a singular focus on sex. According to neuroscientist researcher Margaret McCarthy, 'we cannot know if animals have a perception of their sex, [therefore] the term gender cannot be applied' (McCarthy, 2015, p. 1018). ORWH Director Janine Clayton has similarly suggested that gender is 'less amenable to investigation in preclinical work' (Clayton, 2016b, p. 520). Louise McCullough has stated, 'when I have a little black C57 mouse, they are all exactly the same. So, if you see a difference, it is because of something *you* are doing, whereas in big human populations it can depend on other factors – depression, social factors, compliance' (ACRWH, 2015). Yet the supposed biological purity of animal models relies on a narrow definition of gender that is contradicted by the complex social worlds that laboratory animals reveal.

Consider the following study conducted by pain researcher Jeffrey Mogil (Sorge et al., 2014). Mogil and colleagues discovered that the gender of the experimenter impacted the pain response of lab mice injected with zymosan, an inflammatory agent used to experimentally induce a pain response, measured with the mouse grimace scale. They found that if the observing experimenter in the room was a cisgender man, both female and male mice exhibited a reduction in facial grimacing relative to either a cisgender woman experimenter or no observer at all.[5] Mice had the same inhibited pain response when even a T-shirt worn by a cisgender man was left in the room. The researchers concluded that the response was olfactory and linked to the higher concentration of androgens typically secreted by male bodies. Yet they chose to explain this effect in terms of evolutionary biology, rather than as a dynamic relational effect.

An even more striking example of this biologizing of complex laboratory relations arose during the 2015 SABV panel, when McCullough described her research social isolation and its effects on stroke severity and recovery in lab mice:

> We knew that social isolation is as big of a risk for stroke as is hypertension, and it is as big of a risk for poor recovery from stroke ... If you take two animals and separate them a week before you induce a stroke, their stroke is 50% bigger ... and if you give them the exact same stroke, you leave them together and then separate them, the isolated one dies 30 days later ... *So, that is something very fundamental and very biological.*

McCullough shared this vignette to demonstrate the kinds of phenomena that can be studied in animals but not humans, due to the latter's complex behavioural and social tendencies. Yet in fact, McCullough reveals that animal models can offer key insights into the social dynamics of health – in this instance, the health effects of social isolation. Thus, the mechanisms that some researchers categorise as 'purely' 'biological sex' are very much entangled with the social relations of the lab, a point that historian of science Londa Schiebinger has also emphasised to NIH policymakers: 'these gender differences are precisely the ones that we might mistake for sex differences' (ORWH, 2014b; see also Gungor et al., 2019). In turn, this means that gender – defined in terms of laboratory context – may impact the reproducibility of experiments, purportedly the key motivation for introducing the SABV policy in the first place.

The messy material-discursive entanglement of gender and sex has in fact been raised on numerous occasions during SABV policy discussions. During a 2014 workshop (ORWH, 2014b), neuroscientist Gillian Einstein pushed participants to consider the relevance of gender to animal research. She asked, for example, what new lines of inquiry might open if researchers approached the lab animal's environment 'as a metaphor for the gendered world' of humans? The following discussion ensued involving basic scientist Teresa Woodruff:

> Woodruff: When you metaphorize, do you think of animals that are mammals? … How far do we metaphorize given the two definitions that you've provided us which have to do with environmental interactions? You can say zebra fish have this. So, where are the metaphoritic boundary conditions?
>
> Einstein: I just want to say that first of all, there are fish that definitely have genders that change. So, the protogynous fish …
>
> Audience: They have sex!
>
> Einstein: Their sex changes but there must be something in the interaction of the fact that there is no male.
>
> Audience: They detect that there's no male but that doesn't mean that they have gender.
>
> Einstein: Well, I really think that they have gender in the sense that there is an environment in which they're interacting …
>
> Woodruff: It depends on your definition. The definition of interaction with the environment, if that is gender …
>
> Schiebinger: I think the sex of the fish … it's the sex that changes in reaction to the gender interaction of the group. That's what I would say.
>
> Einstein: Yes, thank you.

Here sex and gender are ultimately revealed as entangled: the sex of the protogynous fish changes in response to gendered group dynamics, but with no clear distinction between the two.

Even so, these policymaking moments constitute agential openings where dominant narratives may be rewritten. A commentary published following the 2014 ORWH workshop describes a range of ways that gender is relevant to animal research (and especially mice), including researcher interactions, housing arrangements, and the differential effects of laboratory 'domestication' on female versus male mice (Figure 3) (Klein et al., 2015). In response to the SABV policy, then, laboratory animals 'kicked back' to reveal the social character of their laboratory world.

Varying multiply

If sex is a so-called biological variable, in what ways does it vary? Proponents of the SABV policy tend to suggest a distinctly binary understanding of sex-linked variation: 'at the most basic level, people – and animals – come in *two forms*: female and male' (Clayton, 2015a, emphasis added). At the conclusion of the 2015 SABV panel, discussant and geneticist David Page presented an artist's rendering of Noah's Ark 'to illustrate the fact that we have all known since childhood: … [that] the commonality across the animal kingdom is the existence of male and female.' Of course, such a claim overlooks the existence of nonbinary variation in both human and non-human species (Fausto-Sterling,

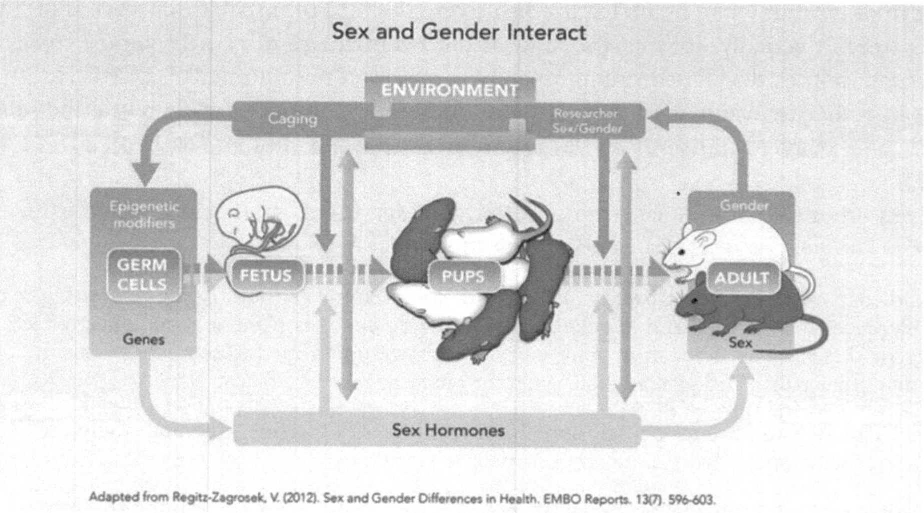

Figure 3. Gender and sex as entangled in animal models (Klein et al., 2015, p. 5257).

2000). Also overlooked is the fact that the trait variation that researchers set out to measure in laboratory animals frequently does not conform to a neat female/male binary.

For example, variation commonly takes the form of *average differences* between females and males but with considerable overlap in distributions (Joel, 2016; Ritz et al., 2014). In a 2016 presentation to the ACRWH, neuroscientist and animal researcher Jill Becker stated that she has come to 'think about sex differences as not being a bimodal distribution but more of a *continuum* … You don't have 'the male phenotype' and 'the female phenotype,' you have the variation between those' (ACRWH, 2016). To illustrate, Becker described the cocaine habits of laboratory rats: female rats choose to consume cocaine over a banana-flavored pellet *more often* than males, but one in six male rats will nevertheless develop a cocaine habit.[6] In other words, the sex differences she observes are not absolute, meaning the sex category assigned to an animal (female or male) does not necessarily predict how it will behave, express a particular trait, or respond to a particular drug (Joel, 2016).

Becker's interventions provide further insight into the complex (and context-specific) ways that sex-linked variation can occur in laboratory animals. She emphasised that in rodent models, for example, it is particularly important to take note of differences in social structure across orders and species:

> [O]ne of the things that people need to be aware of is that the social structure for other species is quite different. Rats are quite different from mice … the mom and the daughters stay with the natal group and the males disperse, [whereas] mice are harem breeders … so the males live with the females in a large group … A valid stress for a rat might not be the same thing as a valid stress for a mouse. (ACRWH, 2014)

On another occasion, Becker emphasised the olfactory nature of relations amongst mice in particular: 'these cues are really important to mice' and therefore impact experimental design. She added, '[a]s we think about rats and mice, we need to think about how they live in *their* world' (ACRWH, 2016). Geneticist Art Arnold similarly shared with policymakers that when he first started studying the bird brain, he discovered that '[his] birds weren't actually obeying the laws of the twentieth century with regard to sexual differentiation as developed predominately in research on mammals' (ACRWH, 2015). That is, rather than universal laws of binary difference, animal models reveal the *multiplicity* of sex-linked traits as they vary from one species to another (Latham, 2017; Pape, 2021).

Even amongst some mice strains, patterns in sex-linked traits can change from one litter to the next, as was discussed during the 2015 SABV panel:

> Audience member: I have been wrestling with something. We found some interesting sex differences in wild type and knockout mice. How do you sort if there is no cohort effect? ... All the progeny come from one pair of each we got from Jackson labs. What if... some other pair could give a whole different outcome?
>
> Art Arnold: You have to look at more litters ... It is really important because there are big litter effects, especially in some strains or some situations.

This suggests that if the goal of the SABV policy is to address the issue of rigor and reproducibility in animal models, it will require more than the mere addition of female models and analysis of results by sex: accounting for observed variation demands intimate knowledge of species-specific, laboratory-specific, or even cohort-specific factors (Eliot & Richardson, 2016).

This, in turn, prompts the question of when and how animal models can inform understandings of human health. After all, the ultimate goal of the SABV mandate is to advance health knowledge – especially as it relates to women, who are deemed directly compromised by the overreliance on male models in animal research (Clayton, 2015b). Here there is an assumed degree of equivalency between human and non-human females: including the latter should advance understanding of 'the normal development of women, and their health and diseases' (ACRWH, 2007). However, in the first meeting of the ACRWH following the SABV policy announcement, neuroscientist Emeran Mayer cautioned against assuming this *a priori*:

> Sex differences are species-dependent ... The sex difference in some trait in a mouse and a rat does not necessarily translate to a sex difference in humans. We've found this in pain [research] many times, to the big surprise of everybody, that one group finds dramatic sex differences in terms of visceral pain in the animals, but we don't see this really in our human patients. (ACRWH, 2014)

Consistent with this insight, during the 2015 SABV panel, speakers emphasised the value of animals as sources of 'bright ideas that *might* be true of humans,' even though 'a mouse is not a human by any stretch of the imagination' (see also Gungor et al., 2019). Thus, the relevance of animal models to humans – women or otherwise – remains an open question. Animals offer at best (and perhaps not even) partial models of sex-linked variation in humans, because of the *multiple*, context-specific, and indeterminate ways that sex varies in practice.

Conclusion: towards response-able animal research

> The ethical questions that we will want to consider are not only about how nonhuman animals are being appropriated for human desires but also about how our desires and our beings are co-constitutively reconfigured as well. (Barad, 2007, pp. 393–394)

I have argued that rule-making practices for biomedical research constitute material-discursive interventions that are implicated in laboratory phenomena and serve not only as *agential cuts* (boundary-drawing moments) but also as *agential openings*: moments of potential response-ability in which human-nonhuman relations might be redrawn (Barad, 2007; Haraway, 2016). In the case of the SABV policy, these practices shed light on the ever-social nature of scientific research and how gender politics become entangled with human-nonhuman relations within the biomedical enterprise. Yet there is a disconnect between SABV policy enactments of sex – as a binary and biological variable that can be studied by the addition of female animals – and what laboratory animals reveal in practice: an indeterminate and multiply varying collection of traits that always exist in relational, context-specific, and dynamic ways (Eliot & Richardson, 2016; Richardson, 2021).

Biomedical researchers appear to simultaneously recognise this complexity yet obscure it, just as NIH policymakers appear to both acknowledge their simplistic policy language and resist adapting the SABV mandate, such as to make room for gender in basic and preclinical research (Clayton, 2016b). As recently as a 2019 meeting of the ACRWH, for example, ORWH representatives emphasised sex as a stand-alone policy focus, despite one committee member urging that 'what we are worrying about with gender in humans is something that we *do* need to worry about in animal research' (ACRWH, 2019). After all, neither rigor and reproducibility nor health will be well served if the key contextual mechanisms that shape experimental outcomes are not given due consideration.

Richardson and colleagues (2015) make a similar point with respect to adverse drug reactions, often promoted by NIH policymakers as a key justification for the SABV policy (Clayton & Collins, 2014). The logic is as follows: women more often experience adverse drug reactions than men, pointing to underlying fundamental biological mechanisms that have been obscured by inattention to sex in basic and preclinical research. Yet as Richardson and colleagues (2015) argue, this disparity might equally be due to polypharmacy (taking multiple drugs at one time) – a behaviour known to be more common in women and a key cause of adverse drug reactions. As in the case of social isolation and stroke recovery, what health and illness mechanisms are excluded from biomedical knowledge-making when the focus is on sex alone, narrowly defined? Animal models might well resist the 'constraints and exclusions' that the SABV mandate seeks to impose on patterns of mattering, but the conversations that *could* be had are nevertheless limited (Barad, 2003, p. 815).

While this article has focused on animal research, cell lines further reveal the unavoidably contextual nature of sex (Ritz, 2017). NIH policymakers originally intended to include cell-based research in the SABV mandate, but were ultimately made to recognise that cell lines cannot be categorised by sex (NIH, 2018). As one cell researcher submitted to the NIH following the announcement of the SABV policy: '[t]ransformed cell lines from a male donor certainly can't be said to 'represent' women, but they shouldn't be understood as 'representing' men either … [I]n vitro research can never account for the totality of sex; at best, it can represent 'aspects of sex'' (NIH, 2014). That is, the contextual (and multidimensional) nature of sex means that it does not simply reside perpetually in a cell, calling into question the favoured line of ORWH policymakers that 'every cell has a sex' (Clayton, 2016b, p. 521).

What would be the practical implications of a reimagined conceptualisation of sex for actual practices of basic and preclinical research? Reflecting on this question, feminist molecular biologist Stacey Ritz has stated:

> The power of an experiment hinges on its ability to simplify and control, yet so many of these dynamic, fluid, and responsive aspects of sex are impossible to control. What does that mean when we're trying to use the power of the experiment to develop a better understanding of how our biology works and how that translates into health outcomes? ... I find it really hard to envision what that could look like, but I'm also really excited about what might be possible in this space. (Pape, Karkazis, Latham, & Ritz, 2020, p. 12).

Feminist biologists are already taking up this challenge, most often in human research (see for example Hyde et al., 2019; Joel, 2016; van Anders, 2012). Under what experimental – and *regulatory* – conditions might animal models be differently engaged to advance understanding of health and illness? And, what kinds of response-abilities might sociologists develop in order to better engage with the nonhuman dimensions of knowledge projects, particularly as they relate to health, difference, and other 'truth' claims (Fullagar, 2017)? By approaching rule-making practices as constituent elements of material-discursive laboratory phenomena, and viewing these through the intra-active lens of feminist posthumanism, sociologists might generate novel answers to the question of 'how differences get made, what gets excluded and how these exclusions matter' (Barad, 2007, p. 32).

Notes

1. The very demarcation of 'human' from 'nonhuman' can be understood as actively produced rather than given (Barad, 2003; Birke, 2010).
2. The reliance on male models even occurs in research on conditions that are more prevalent in women, such as stroke, anxiety and depression. A small number of fields, such as reproduction and immunology, have a 'female bias' (Zucker & Beery, 2010).
3. Note, too, the slippage from nonhuman to human in Colbert's account.
4. The authors attribute male variance to dominance hierarchies, which can activate a physiological response in both dominant and subordinate cage mates.
5. The researchers found a similar 'male observer' effect in laboratory rats.
6. As Becker herself acknowledged, extrapolating findings on addiction from laboratory mice to humans is complicated, given the significant role of trauma in human addiction habits (ACRWH, 2016).

Acknowledgement

I am grateful to Steve Epstein, Myra Marx Ferree, and Joan Fujimura for their extensive guidance throughout this project. I also thank the reviewers and guest editors of this special issue for their constructive and supportive comments. This research was supported by a Doctoral Dissertation Research Improvement Grant from the National Science Foundation in the United States (Award Number 1849234). Correspondence concerning this manuscript should be addressed to Madeleine Pape, Quartier UNIL-Centre, Bâtiment Synathlon, University of Lausanne, Switzerland; E-mail: madeleine.pape@unil.ch.

Disclosure statement

No potential conflict of interest was reported by the author(s).

Funding

This work was supported by Division of Social and Economic Sciences: [Grant Number 1849234].

ORCID

Madeleine Pape http://orcid.org/0000-0002-8075-5934

References

ACRWH. (2014). 38th ACRWH Meeting (24 September). Videocast. Retrieved from https://videocast.nih.gov/summary.asp?Live=14687&bhcp=1.

ACRWH. (2015). 40th ACRWH Meeting (20 October). Videocast. Retrieved from https://videocast.nih.gov/summary.asp?Live=15589&bhcp=1.

ACRWH. (2016). 41st ACRWH Meeting (19 April). Videocast. Retrieved from https://videocast.nih.gov/summary.asp?Live=18490&bhcp=1.

ACRWH. (2019). 49th ACRWH Meeting (23 October). Videocast. Retrieved from https://videocast.nih.gov/summary.asp?Live=34443&bhcp=1.

ACRWH (Advisory Committee for Research on Women's Health). (2007). Minutes of the 26th ACRWH Meeting (23 October).

Barad, K. (2003). Posthumanist performativity: Toward an understanding of how matter comes to matter. *Signs: Journal of Women in Culture and Society*, *28*(3), 801–831.

Barad, K. (2007). *Meeting the universe halfway: Quantum physics and the entanglement of matter and meaning*. Durham, NC: Duke University Press.

Begley, C., & Ellis, L. M. (2012). Raise standards for preclinical cancer research. *Nature*, *483*, 51–533.

Birke, L. (2010). Structuring relationships: On science, feminism and non-human animals. *Feminism & Psychology*, *20*(3), 337–349.

Birke, L., Bryld, M., & Lykke, N. (2004). Animal performances: An exploration of intersections between feminist science studies and studies of human/animal relationships. *Feminist Theory*, *5*(2), 167–183.

Bleier, R. (1984). *Science and gender: A critique of biology and its theories on women*. New York: Pergamon.

Brooks, C. E., & Clayton, J. (2016). Sex/gender influences on the nervous system: Basic steps toward clinical progress. *Journal of Neuroscience Research*, *95*(1–2), 14–16.

Callon, M. (1984). Some elements of a sociology of translation: Domestication of the scallops and the fishermen of St brieuc Bay. *The Sociological Review*, *32*(1), 196–233.

Callon, M., & Law, J. (1997). After the individual in society: Lessons on collectivity from science, technology and society. *The Canadian Journal of Sociology*, *22*(2), 165–182.

Clayton, J. A. (2015a). Considering sex as a biological variable in NIH-funded preclinical research. Letter from the Director, National Institute of Arthritis and Musculoskeletal and Skin Diseases. 20 August 2015. Retrieved from: https://www.niams.nih.gov/about/about-the-director/letter/considering-sex-biological-variable-nih-funded-preclinical-research

Clayton, J. A. (2015b) Happy 25th birthday, ORWH! Director's message, 31 October 2015. Retrieved from: https://orwh.od.nih.gov/about/director/messages/orwh-anniversary

Clayton, J. A. (2016a). Sex as a biological variable: A step toward stronger science, better health. Director's Messages, 1 February. Retrieved from https://orwh.od.nih.gov/about/director/messages/sex-biological-variable.

Clayton, J. A. (2016b). Studying both sexes: A guiding principle for biomedicine. *FASEB*, *30*(2), 519–524.

Clayton, J. A., & Collins, F. S. (2014). Policy: NIH to balance sex in cell and animal studies. *Nature*, *509*(7500), 282–283.

Colbert Report, The. (2014). Co-ed lab rats. 19 May 2014. Retrieved from http://www.cc.com/video-clips/el90zp/the-colbert-report-co-ed-lab-rats.

Collins, F. S., & Tabak, L. A. (2014). NIH plans to enhance reproducibility. *Nature, 505*(7485), 612–613.

Eliot, L., & Richardson, S. S. (2016). Sex in context: Limitations of animal studies for addressing human sex/gender neurobehavioral health disparities. *Journal of Neuroscience, 36*(47), 11823–11830.

Epstein, S. (2007). *Inclusion: The politics of difference in medical research.* Chicago: University of Chicago Press.

Fausto-Sterling, A. (2000). *Sexing the body: Gender politics and the construction of sexuality.* New York: Basic Books.

Frickel, S., Gibbon, S., et al. (2009). Undone science: Charting social movement and civil society challenges to research agenda setting. *Science, Technology, & Human Values, 35*(4), 444–473.

Fujimura, J. (2006). Sex genes: A critical sociomaterial approach to the politics and molecular genetics of sex determination. *Signs, 32*(1), 49–82.

Fullagar, S. (2017). Post-qualitative inquiry and the new materialist turn: Implications for sport, health and physical culture research. *Qualitative Research in Sport, Exercise and Health, 9*(2), 247–257.

Gendered Innovations. (2020). Sex and gender analysis policies of major granting agencies. Retrieved from http://genderedinnovations.stanford.edu/sex-and-gender-analysis-policies-major-granting-agencies.html.

Gungor, N. Z., Duchesne, A., & Bluhm, R. (2019). A conversation around the integration of sex and gender when modeling aspects of fear, anxiety, and PTSD in animals. *S&F Online, 15*, 2.

Haraway, D. (1988). Situated knowledges: The science question in feminism and the privilege of partial perspective. *Feminist Studies, 14*(3), 575–599.

Haraway, D. (2016). *Staying with the trouble: Making kin in the Chthulucene.* Durham, NC: Duke University Press.

Hess, D. J. (2004). Medical modernisation, scientific research fields and the epistemic politics of health social movements. *Sociology of Health & Illness, 26*(6), 695–709.

Hyde, J. S., Bigler, R. S., et al. (2019). The future of sex and gender in psychology: Five challenges to the gender binary. *American Psychologist, 74*(2), 171–193.

Jasanoff, S. (2005). *Designs on nature: Science and democracy in Europe and the United States.* Princeton, NJ: Princeton University Press.

Joel, D. (2016). VIII. Captured in terminology: Sex, sex categories, and sex differences. *Feminism & Psychology, 26*(3), 335–345.

Jordan-Young, R. M. (2012). *Brain storm: The flaws in the science of sex differences.* Cambridge, MA: Harvard University Press.

Jordan-Young, R. M., & Karkazis, K. (2019). *Testosterone: An unauthorized biography.* Cambridge, MA: Harvard University Press.

Karkazis, K. (2019). The misuses of 'biological sex.'. *The Lancet, 394*(10212), 1898–1899.

Keller, E. F. (1985). *Reflections on gender and science.* New Haven: Yale University Press.

Klein, S. L., Schiebinger, L., et al. (2015). Opinion: Sex inclusion in basic research drives discovery. *PNAS, 112*(17), 5257–5258.

Krieger, N. (2003). Gender, sexes, and health: What are the connections – and why does it matter? *International Journal of Epidemiology, 32*(4), 652–657.

Latham, J. R. (2017). (Re)making sex: A praxiography of the gender clinic. *Feminist Theory, 18*(2), 177–204.

Latour, B. (2000). When things strike back: A possible contribution of 'science studies' to the social sciences. *British Journal of Sociology, 51*(1), 107–123.

Latour, B. (2005). *Reassembling the social: An introduction to actor-network theory.* New York: Oxford University Press.

Martin, E. (1991). The egg and the sperm. *Signs, 16*, 485–501.

McCarthy, M. (2015). Incorporating sex as a variable in preclinical neuropsychiatric research. *Schizophrenia Bulletin, 41*(5), 1016–1020.

National Institutes of Health (NIH). (2014). Request for Information (RFI): Consideration of Sex as a Biological Variable in Biomedical Research. Notice Number: NOT-OD-14-128.

NIH. (2015). Enhancing reproducibility through rigor and transparency. NIH notice number: NOT-OD-15-103. Retrieved from https://grants.nih.gov/grants/guide/notice-files/not-od-15-103.html.

NIH. (2018). Frequently asked questions (FAQs): Rigor and reproducibility. Retrieved from https://grants.nih.gov/faqs#/rigor-and-reproducibility.htm?anchor=question54422.

Office of Research on Women's Health (ORWH). (2014a). *Methods and Techniques for Integrating the Biological Variable Sex into Preclinical Research*. Report. Bethesda, MD: Office of Research on Women's Health, National Institutes of Health.

ORWH. (2014b). Methods and Techniques for Integrating the Biological Variable Sex into Preclinical Research, October 20. Videocast. Retrieved from https://videocast.nih.gov/watch=14501.

Pape, M. (2021). Co-production, multiplied: Enactments of sex as a biological variable in U. S. biomedicine. *Social Studies of Science*, *51*(3), 339–363.

Pape, M., Karkazis, K., Latham, J. R., & Ritz, S. (2020). Lab meeting: Resisting and remaking sex in the petri dish, the clinic, and on the track. *Catalyst: Feminism, Theory, Technoscience*, *6*(2), 1–18.

Prendergast, B. J., Onishi, K. G., & Zucker, I. (2014). Female mice liberated for inclusion in neuroscience and biomedical research. *Neuroscience & Behavioral Reviews*, *40*, 1–5.

Richardson, S. (2013). *Sex itself: The search for male and female in the human genome*. Chicago: University of Chicago Press.

Richardson, S. (2021). Sex contextualism. Unpublished manuscript.

Richardson, S. S., Reiches, M., et al. (2015). Focus on preclinical sex differences will not address women's and men's health disparities. *Proceedings of the National Academy of Sciences*, *112* (44), 13419–13420.

Ritz, S. A. (2017). Complexities of addressing sex in cell culture research. *Signs*, *42*(2), 307–327.

Ritz, S. A., Antle, D. M., et al. (2014). First steps for integrating sex and gender considerations into basic experimental biomedical research. *The FASEB Journal*, *28*(1), 4–13.

Society for Women's Health Research (SWHR). (2015). SWHR applauds NIH's new inclusion of sex as a biological variable. Retrieved from htps://swhr.org/swhr-applauds-nihs-new-inclusion-of-sex-as-a-biological-variable/.

Sorge, R. E., Martin, L. J., et al. (2014). Olfactory exposure to males, including men, causes stress and related analgesia in rodents. *Nature Methods*, *11*, 629–632.

Springer, K. W., Stellman, J. M., & Jordan-Young, R. M. (2012). Beyond a catalogue of differences. *Social Science & Medicine*, *74*(11), 1817–1824.

Terry, J. (2000). "Unnatural acts" in nature: The scientific fascination with queer animals. *GLQ: A Journal of Lesbian and Gay Studies*, *6*(2), 151–193.

van Anders, S. (2012). Testosterone and sexual desire in healthy women and men. *Archives of Sexual Behavior*, *41*(6), 1471–1484.

Zucker, I., & Beery, A. K. (2010). Males still dominate animal studies. *Nature*, *465*(7299), 690.

A posthuman decentring of person-centred care

Barbara E. Gibson, Joanna K. Fadyl, Gareth Terry, Kate Waterworth, Donya Mosleh and Nicola M. Kayes

ABSTRACT

In this paper, we examine person-centred care through a Deleuzian posthuman lens with the aim of exploring what becomes possible when the concepts of both person and care are *de-centred*. We do so through a consideration of the sets of relations that produce 'the client' in health care contexts. Our analysis maps particular entangled material-semiotic forces producing 'M/michael', a young man with a diagnosis of Duchenne muscular dystrophy, within a rehabilitation clinic. Drawing on Deleuzian notions of *assemblage*, *affect*, and *becoming* we explore 'person-care' as an active production that dynamically enacts persons-as-clients through clinical arrangements. Persons are thus reconceptualised in terms of locally produced subject positions and their care relations, rather than pre-existing beings who can be 'centred' within health services. Paradoxically, by de-centring persons and care, we work to conjure ways to strengthen the aspirations of person centredness to humanise health practices. In doing so, we consider different possibilities for re-imagining clinical work and contribute to debates regarding how healthcare conceptualises and addresses disability, health, and wellbeing. We suggest that such posthuman analyses can open up new ways of understanding and re/forming healthcare.

Humanist person-centred care within biomedicine: competing priorities

Person-centred care (PCC) has sought to revolutionise biomedical healthcare by re-orienting clinical work to caring for people rather than curing pathology (Leplege et al., 2007). While there are multiple and sometimes competing articulations of PCC, all aim to address the suppression of patient voices, support patient preferences and choices, and orient practices to their unique circumstances. Grounded in notions of 'respect for persons', more sophisticated strands of PCC (e.g. family-centred care, relationship-centred care) extend beyond the individual to attend to the needs of all persons involved, i.e. clinicians, patients and significant others, and signal a move away from 'patient'-centred care. PCC and its variants work to ensure care is meaningfully addressing patient needs and wants, ensuring respectful relationships, mitigating paternalism, and considering how the system supports or constrains these goals. PCC thus has highly laudable goals and has transformed how healthcare is understood and delivered. Despite these changes, problems persist in how PCC is operationalised by health systems, institutions, and individual practitioners. In this paper, we approach these challenges using posthuman 'experimentation', employing Deleuzian concepts to explore what becomes possible when notions of both person and care are *de-centred.*

PCC competes with other powerful forces and ideas that also significantly shape health practices and delivery. These include the persistence of biomedical/pathological framings of health and illness, positivist and reductive notions of the body as a machine, and the imposition of 'evidence-based practice' that venerates the randomised controlled trial over all other forms of knowledge production (Holmes, Murray, Perron, & Rail, 2006). Within medicine, objective assessment 'findings' are the core of clinical reasoning processes, which are designed to logically interpret data towards determining a diagnosis and treatment plan based on 'best evidence'. Moreover, with increasing interest in machine learning, data-driven decision making tends towards reducing 'persons' to a series of data points, and 'care' to increasingly standardised sets of algorithmic procedures (Holford, 2020). Keeping persons centred is thus difficult work within these competing imperatives.

The evolution of PCC has seen it increasingly align with biomedical and managerial approaches to care. The dominance of evidence-based practice and the enthusiasm for data-driven management manifests in the operationalisation of PCC in the form of checklists, questionnaires, and measures that reduce delivery and evaluation of care to a set of statistically analyzable numbers (Edvardsson & Innes, 2010). This can be seen in articulations of PCC that stress the development of quality indicators, measurable frameworks, and organisational performance (Guastello & Jay, 2019). While our intention is not to suggest these approaches are irredeemable or do nothing to achieve improvements in individualised care, we argue that the core aims of PCC may be compromised when increasing aligned with the systematisation of healthcare delivery.

Despite the apparent differences between positivist biomedicine and humanist PCC, they nevertheless share common conceptions of persons as pre-formed agents, holding subjective viewpoints and preferences, and acting as autonomous beings in the world. Each approach may assign different degrees of value to 'the patient's voice', but they agree that individuals 'hold' opinions and have personal priorities that can be elicited. But there are other ways of understanding subjects and subjectivities that we suggest may be mobilised to assist PCC to realise its aspirations. Our aim in the paper is to engage in posthuman experimentation oriented to 'producing different knowledge and producing knowledge differently' (Monforte & Smith, 2021, p. 652) in order to inspire creative approaches to thinking and doing PCC. Our team is comprised of senior and junior scholars from varied social locations and disciplines that include psychology, disability studies, bioethics, rehabilitation, and health sciences. Some of us work primarily in critical and/or posthuman spaces, others in PCC and/or rehabilitation. We are/ have been 'patients', 'clinicians' and 'parents', and a host of other subject positions. In drawing on posthuman scholarship to rethink the person in healthcare, we aim to de-centre PCC- not to replace it or derail it, but to help it to thrive.

In what follows, we provide a Deleuzian de-centring of 'persons' and 'care' by working through various arrangements of objects and subjects implicated in producing 'M/

michael' as 'patient with muscular dystrophy' within the context of a rehabilitation clinic. We then conclude with a discussion of the implications of de-centred person-care for informing the aims of PCC.

Becoming persons

We begin by introducing some key tenets of our posthuman approach and the Deleuzian concepts we employ. Deleuze's writings, and those with his collaborator Guattari, continue to exert considerable influence across fields of inquiry, including healthcare scholarship where it intersects with science and technology studies, disability studies, and the sociology of health (e.g. Blume, Galis, & Pineda, 2014; Buse, Martin, & Nettleton, 2018; Moser, 2006). While there are multiple strands of posthuman theory, all challenge the humanist project, scientific proceduralism, and the centrality of Western knowledge and truth (Carlson, Wells, Mark, & Sandoval, 2021).

Contra prevailing humanist understandings of humans as self-contained, closed, and autonomous subjects, our posthuman approach considers the radical openness of people and bodies. Subjects are reconfigured as in a continual state of flux, neither encased by skin and organs nor defined by static binary categorisations, such as disabled/able-bodied, male/female, person/thing, or myself/other (Gibson, 2006; Massumi, 1992). The defining features of the human condition – e.g. agency, subjectivity, identity, judgment, values, and bodies – are no longer viewed as stable properties of a contained self but rather as *outcomes* of generative processes (Andrews & Duff, 2019). In other words, humans and their capacities are reconceived as continually being made and unmade across different encounters. This decentring of the autonomous subject creates space for analyzing the interactions between human and non-human entities without privileging (or 'centring') one over the other.

The notion that no/thing is static but always in constant production runs across Deleuze's work. A subject for Deleuze is re-imagined as perpetual *becoming* through an open system of *assemblages* – as opposed to a closed and static 'subject' – that is continually reconfigured. *Assemblage* is Deleuze and Guattari's (1987) term to characterise the constantly shifting connectivities between heterogeneous material-semiotic forces and entities, including but not limited to bodies, social meanings, emotions, objects, places, and technologies. Each of these entities or 'singularities' are themselves continually composed and recomposed. Thus, there are no self-contained parts that make up an assemblage, but rather assemblages are dynamic and temporary, coming-together in specific arrangements to produce objects and subjects that have the appearance of permanence and solidity. Assemblages can be thought of as 'machines' that can be 'plugged in' to other machines that do things in the world (Deleuze & Guattari, 1987). Human and other assemblages are thus neither stable or closed systems, but temporary entanglements that continually compose, decompose, and recompose, forming different machinic assemblages with other material-semiotic forces that produce different capacities. Persons in such a formulation are particular assemblages produced through intersecting animate sensibilities and materialities. Within such a configuration, the imagined autonomous persons of PCC are radically reconfigured. Not simply an exercise in alternative description, our focus on mapping dynamic assemblages in the paper works to enact an open and affirmative person-care ethics. To do so we need to briefly sketch two related Deleuzian concepts: becoming and desire.

Becoming expresses Deleuze and Guatarri's process ontology wherein subjects as not only in flux but with a directionality that resists becoming fixed or 'territorialized'. Assemblages coalesce through capacities of assembled relations to affect or be affected. This capacity is becoming, i.e. a change of state or relations which may be physical, biological, psychological, social, political, or emotional (Fox & Alldred, 2017). As Braidotti (2013) notes, becoming-machines 'stand for radical relationality and delight as well as productivity' (p. 92). Becoming is thus always an affirmative movement towards something but not in a temporal sense of futurity. As a force of production, becoming marks the unceasing mobility of collective life: 'A kind of order or apparent progressions can be established for the segments of becoming in which we find ourselves; becoming-woman, becoming-child, becoming-animal, – vegetable, or mineral; becomings – molecular of all kinds, becoming-particles' (Deleuze & Guattari, 1987, p. 272). Becoming expresses a nonlinearity that nevertheless has directionality in the sense that it escapes or breaks away from that which has previously sought to contain it, resisting and reconstituting borders.

Deleuze and Guattari (1987) see the individuation of the subject as limiting *desire*. Desire is not a want or a compulsion to address a lack of something but rather, it is a positive and productive force (*puissance*) of becoming. Linked with the concept of *affect*, desire is the ability to affect and to be affected, to form emergent unities (assemblages) that retain the heterogeneity of their components (Deleuze, 1978). Affective forces amplify and compel awareness, movements, thoughts, or expressions and are transmittable within and between bodies, things, and environments (Shouse, 2005). Emotions/ideas/thoughts are related to affect but are produced through relations rather than belonging to individuals. Moreover, while concepts like affect, becoming and desire have a consistency in Deleuzian analysis, they do not have an essential identity (Smith, 2020). Rather than a problem, the becoming of concepts opens thought to creative possibilities or affirmative 'lines of flight'. The unthought becomes thinkable.

What does this mean for PCC? We begin by rejecting the notion of a care encounter occurring between autonomous 'persons' within a static healthcare 'setting' and according to hierarchical (Deleuze might say 'arborescent') divisions of micro/meso/macro 'contexts'. In doing so, we endeavour to move beyond a critique of the actual (what is, or more precisely, what is ceasing to be) to creative actualisation of the virtual (the possible processes of becoming) (Braidotti, 2019). De-centred care in our exploration is an affective and affirmative production, a shifting 'becoming person-care assemblage' that is made by and responds to a set of relations with multiple effects that open opportunities.

Becoming – M/michael

To reconsider person-care, we map becoming person-care assemblages with their compositions, flows, and entanglements across time–space events. Our analysis takes as its entry point a young man named 'Michael' who participated in an earlier observational study exploring children's rehabilitation care practices (Abrams, Setchell, Thille, Mistry, & Gibson, 2019; Setchell et al., 2018). In PCC, Michael would be 'the client' (or patient) around whom care would be centred, considering how the values, perspectives and needs of all 'persons' in a clinical care encounter could be respected. In our analysis, Michael is understood as a conglomeration of forces that produce the enduring subject position that is recognised as Michael but continually changes in different iterations (different 'michaels') as he moves through the world. We deliberately switch to a lower case 'm' here to signal there is no essential 'Michael' but several possible iterations, several michaels, none of which can be labelled 'him' (Michael self-identified as male/man). Thus, in the paper we use the upper case to refer to the Michael of the clinic, lower case for becoming-michael, and M/michael when these positions overlap.

We first describe M/michael in somewhat conventional terms of a humanist 'case' recognising that in so doing we produce a particular michael assemblage (casing the case, c.f. Sandelowski, 2011). We deliberately use this familiar (in healthcare) style of presentation to examine the kinds of subjects that are produced in representation, recognising that we as authors are implicated in these productions, and that the case does not pre-exist but is produced as part of a research assemblage (Fox & Alldred, 2018). We then use the case as a point of departure for decentring Michael-as-person by re-assembling the case through two different re-composing experiments: becoming-chair and becoming-death/life. Writing and representing posthuman subjects is a tricky business but here we have chosen to employ 'becoming' as a shorthand modifier for the decentred assemblages that we map, recognising that we risk a reductive reading of becoming which we return to below. Each iteration draws from a set of observation notes produced in a Canadian study examining clinical practices with a children's rehabilitation team, the details of which have been published elsewhere (Setchell et al., 2018).

'Michael' as research case

Michael (all names are pseudonyms) was a 16-year-old in grade 10 at a Canadian high school. At the age of five, he was diagnosed with Duchenne muscular dystrophy (DMD). DMD is described in medicine as a life-limiting condition characterised by progressive muscle weakness which leads to a loss of function and mobility, and eventual respiratory failure. Life expectancy ranges between 25 and 40 years but is highly uncertain (Landfeldt et al., 2020). Michael lived at home with his mum, dad and older brother. His mum, Jee, did most of Michael's personal care (bathing, dressing, etc.). Michael spent much of his spare time watching anime which he said was his 'favourite thing to do'. He started using a manual wheelchair at age 12, but it was increasingly difficult to self-propel and the family had recently purchased a power chair that Michael was using at school. At home he used a wheeled office chair that Jee pushed for him. Members of his clinical team expressed concern with Michael's continued 'reliance on Mum' for mobility and transfers and the effects this had on her physically, psychologically, and socially.

Michael attended an outpatient medical clinic at a children's rehabilitation hospital every four months, usually with Jee. During these appointments, the family would sit in a clinic room while six to eight multidisciplinary clinicians took turns coming in to conduct various medical assessments, and to discuss challenges, treatments, and other supports. The following observation notes were made over the course of two clinic visits. Some of the details have been altered to protect confidentiality:

> When the physiotherapist (PT) asked how well the office chair was working for the family, Jee said 'I am not completely happy with the chair, but it's what Michael wants'. She added that she was looking into getting Michael a better manual chair to use around the house, so that 'he can be more independent and not have to always call me for help'. When the PT agreed that this was a great idea, Michael turned to his mum (Jee) and slowly said 'I don't want it. I won't use it'. The PT expressed concern with his use of the office chair, particularly in terms of joint alignment issues and an increased risk of falling, especially during transfers [the office chair does not have brakes]. Jee and the PT tried to persuade Michael that using the more supportive wheelchair would 'be better for him'. Michael continued to refuse. The PT reiterated the benefits of using the manual chair, such as moving himself around the house when he wanted something. She then asked him, 'is that important to you?' Michael shook his head and responded, 'no'. Jee, expressed frustration, and asked Michael if he just wanted her to 'continue to do everything' for him, to which he replied, 'yes'. The PT and the social worker offered to help the family apply for funding to buy an adjustable desk. Michael refused, and said, 'I don't see the point'. When asked why, he said with annoyance, 'because I don't want to'. Jee suggested the only reason he did not want to try a new manual chair in the home was because he 'won't be like everyone else'. She added that when the family goes out to a restaurant, Michael sits in the restaurant chairs and gets her place his wheelchair out of sight. …

At a later visit to the clinic, a recreational therapist talked to the family about an employment mentorship program:

> The therapist turned to Michael and said, 'I remember you were interested in employment, right?' Michael did not respond. The therapist waited for a moment. She then asked, 'Not interested?' Michael slowly said, 'Not really' and looked away. Jee, sounding annoyed, asked 'Why not? This mentor could really help you. You're going to be an adult soon!' The therapist waited for Michael to reply but he did not. She then turned to Jee and said he would not be eligible to register again for another six months, but in the meantime, he could think about it. Jee nodded and asked who they needed to contact to register, but Michael said to her with annoyance, 'Why? I won't change my mind'.

Posthumanist re-composings

The case reveals the mechanisms by which care practices and persons are enacted through entangled material-semiotic forces. The different forms of care in a clinic can be understood as 'events', that is, they are made and unmade through entwined human and non-human, animate and inanimate, material and abstract forces. The diagnosis of DMD catalyzes different ways of knowing and doing of michael and family. The 'client', 'Mum', and the 'client's family' are produced as particular kinds of persons in PCC through biomedical logics – assessments to identify problems, treatments to enhance capacities, psychosocial and material supports, and discourses of child development, independence, biophysical decline, hope etc. Clinicians employ certain treatments, suggestions, 'patient education', and approaches which draw on particular dominant logics and discourses embedded in medicine; and work to particularise options and solutions to child and family capacities, life circumstances, and stated preferences (Mol, 2008). In this, they occupy subject positions of responsible clinicians who perform in accordance with the entangled webs of knowledges, practices, values, temporal rhythms, and conventions that permeate clinic spaces and extend into the social worlds of families and diagnosed children. Interacting forces, including the powerful imperatives of biomedicine, actively produce different forms of care, which then work to reinforce, or for Deleuze and Guattari, 'territorialize', certain ideas and ways of being while negating others. Thus 'persons' and 'care' are relational and temporary productions enacted through clinical events forming person-care assemblages that serve particular interests and not others.

A clinic visit entangles with other events to re/produce michael-with-DMD. Michael's refusals to engage in conversation or accept clinical advice differentially produce becoming-michael. Becoming-michael is an affirmative expression of desire, a line of flight that resists capture by the forces that conspire to territorialise a client-subject. In the encounter described above, M/michael enacts 'acceptable' forms of resistance without having to articulate/examine/know the range of internal and external forces that drive choices, i.e. he shrugs, says no, and/or does not engage without ever fully articulating a rationale or explanation. These gestures disrupt the clinical assemblage, becoming something other than client-with-DMD (Abrams & Gibson, 2017; Callon & Rabeharisoa, 2004). Refusals to use a wheelchair act against an imposed identity in a world where to be marked as disabled is to '*dys*appear' (Leder, 1990), that is, to appear as different in a negative register. Elsewhere we have suggested that the social practices and rhetorics that surround childhood disability draw on and sustain ideas of disability as tragedy, compelling a host of activities oriented to achieving or approximate normalcy: normal bodies, normal development, normal social roles, and normal function (Gibson, 2014). These forces are implicated in clinical work but also in family and social life where subjects are produced through the doings of everyday life. The only rationale for refusing the wheelchair is offered by Jee because he 'won't be like everyone else'. Without words, this rationale is silently rejected in the clinical space as not good enough. Michael never articulates this reason or any other. In his resistance, he becomes both normal and different – in different ways in different spaces and renderings. Becoming-michael thus unfolds along affirmative trajectories, decentring PCC and 'client-with-DMD' by resisting the logics of the clinic. He becomes otherwise: A teenager who sits in regular chairs. Both banal and radical, this becoming-chair-body-michael, as we explore below, enacts desire – collectively reworlding the clinic space by 'processing negativity and producing affirmation' (Braidotti, 2019, p. 51).

The discourses of loss, decline, death, and what-to-do are integral to the co-productions of person-care and their particular forms. The assumed 'tragedy' of loss hangs over the clinic encounter. Michael is getting weaker, more impaired, he will die young. This is too difficult to speak about and yet it is present in talk of risks of the office chair, the need for a new chair. The affective weight of decline co-mingles with clinical imperatives to 'inform and educate the patient' – Life will be better if/when you relent. An unspoken principle of shared decision-making shapes clinical practices. This too is a force of production. Listening to the client's articulated preferences is an integral part of PCC. Conciliatory gestures and comments are made. 'Is that important to you?' Discomfort circulates through the assemblage as emotive forces weigh in and on. They set aside the discussion. A mix of emotions such as fear (of humiliation, of decline) and anger (at insistent adults) conspire to produce [michael's] resistance and [adults'] insistence. This was evident in facial expressions, body language, speech rhythms and tone which became more apparent as the visit progressed. Emotions are productive, but also packaged in particular ways to explain and manage them: Not included in our excerpt was a moment when a clinician asked if Michael was 'depressed'. Medicalisation essentialises, controls, and diminishes the significance of feelings which are explained away through a potential diagnosis and form the explanation for 'non-compliance'. M/michael 'takes' a position as resister. But did he 'choose' this position? Did clinicians and 'Mum'/Jee decide their roles? The emotions, rhetoric, expectations, stigma, identities, responsibility, biological decline, weight, mum, and michael intermingle to produce entreatments and resistance: Please? No!

The decentred person-care that we propose works against the centring of individuals to consider care doings, that is, how persons and care are made within healthcare processes, and what is made to matter. Instead of individuals, we consider the *intra*-acting (Barad, 2003) forces that produce assemblages and the possibilities for reimagined person-care. These forces and assemblages are many including emotions, actions, stigma, personal commitments, compliance, resistance, hope etc. These are not the intended outcomes of human(ist) interventions but the results of coalescing forces that conspire to produce particular worlds that have effects on living and dying. De-centred analysis thus maps the making of material lives and circumstances. What assemblages enable a better life? Who is involved in asking and answering this question? How do clinical events and assemblages flow over other life events and relations?

Experiment: becoming-chair

An appreciation of de-centring is aided by moving beyond mapping persons and choices to re-considering the materialities that we have alluded to above. We thus map a different assemblage (map the assemblage differently) – that of the becoming-chair. Becoming-michael is enacted in the production of becoming-chair (hereafter 'chair'), but we suggest that neither precedes their coming together, nor can they be understood as distinct entities. Chair does not 'contain' michael but is rather an expression of michael and of chair: becoming-chair-body-michael (demonstrating the limits of categories and language). With this in mind we case-the-case as assemblage.

Chair co-resides in michael's home. It usually rests beside a desk and was manufactured as an 'office' chair. As such it has particular features: adjustable height, wheels, removable armrests. It can be made to fit different human bodies, to enable deskwork. It is made of sturdy metal, plastic, and upholstery designed for frequent use. Chair is assembled from components and imbued with meanings of design-for-purpose uses. It evokes affection and feelings of ownership (my chair) and trepidation (unsafe chair). It forms assemblages with desk, floor, computer, bodies, preferences, emotions, tasks, values etc. It invites work-sitting but of course, it affords other uses: a dog curling up, a child's spinning play, an unstable standing platform to change a light bulb.

Becoming-chair-body-michael (hereafter body-chair) forms an anime assemblage with a computer which produces pleasure. Along another line, the pleasure assemblage produces body-chair of a particular type: the subject position of the chair. The assemblage is thus an enacted doing. It does and makes many things and then it splits apart, components plugging into other components to do and make otherwise. Body-chair fits under the desk enabling the viewing of anime on a computer screen, becoming with online community. Forces of hunger or an urge to urinate affect a break. This is a break from a task but also a break in the assemblage. The body speaks. Body-chair connects with becoming-jee and together they move to another room, incorporating other objects, to form new assemblages, actions, affects.

The virtual life afforded by anime is constructed in clinic and family life as 'problem' within which chair is complicit but, at the same time, body-chair as a process is an affirmative act of becoming otherwise. Body-chair enacts pleasure within virtual spaces that are both grounded in and reconfigure the materiality of body and chair, actualising the virtual through desire, becoming dispersed. The chair-anime assemblage entangles with masculinised teenage spaces that produce their own logics. Body-chair does not escape lines of gender, age, class, or race, but is complicit in making and unmaking them. Chair with (and without) becoming-michael is thus productive of and produced through the micro-affective politics of the assemblages it forms. It enters into and makes relations that compel actions and have consequences.

In clinical assemblages, biomedical surveillance produces *at-risk* body-chair. The latter provokes anxieties enacting different subject positions in the clinic: The client's body may be damaged (clinician), the mum is overworked (clinician and parent), chair may be taken away (client), 'Am I a bad mum?' (parent), 'I am not properly educating this family' (clinician), 'I am afraid of what happens next' (client). In the entangled clinical event, body-chair is rationalised according to clinic logics and imperatives of safety. It is a path to normalcy, to be 'like everyone else'. These semiotic forces position body-chair as problem and it is placed into peril. Body-chair works to survive not through mobilising other logics but through affective utterances: 'Because I don't want to'. Such talk entangles desire, disrupting the logics of the clinic and the rhetoric of PCC toward an affirmative becoming of doing DMD otherwise. It is a line of flight – plugging in differently, refusing to play the game of 'clinical question-rational response' that cannot be won. Chair-body-michael continues becoming.

Interlude: care-full caring

The concept of 'care' in the provision of health and social services has often been viewed with suspicion. In relation to disabled people and others, so-called 'caring relationships' have resulted in significant harms, including physical, sexual, and emotional abuse (Saxton et al., 2001). Care scholarship has often focused on developing a care ethic that could address the implied paternalism in service provision oriented to enabling more equitable care relationships. However, these attempts are delimited by humanist ideals of choice, autonomy, and self-determination and they may obscure the significance of the affective relations at play in care encounters that PCC works to address. Posthumanist scholars have proposed the notion of 'care-full' care enacted through diverse and open intra-active care assemblages that support becoming (Fullagar, O'Brien, & Pavlidis, 2019).

Our posthuman approach to care-full care aligns with Fritsch's (2010) relational ethics of intercorporeality which posits that it is 'through becoming in-the-world-with-others … that we can begin to conceptualize care' in beneficial ways (p. 3). The different forms of care in clinic encounters can be understood in terms of entangled human, non-human, material, and abstract forces co-mingling to produce different forms of person-care. In de-centring the person, we have rejected the notion of individuated agents engaged in the transaction of giving and receiving care. Instead, we suggest that person-care is dynamically produced through relational assemblages. This approach forces an examination of the ways in which subject positions (and bodies) are produced in particular configurations. Thinking through the relations and extensions of caring (desiring) bodies that exceed their autonomous containment is not simply to point out the ways in which everyone in the care relation is 'interdependent'. Rather, it problematises the separation of giver and receiver, acknowledges that more than individual human agency is at play, and demonstrates the active production of becoming. We explore these ideas further below, but first map a second experiment.

Experiment: becoming-death/life

We move now to consider temporalities of DMD and how 'the client with degenerative disease' is varyingly constituted across socio-temporal spaces in relation to decline and death. Death myriad differs from an office chair but is similar in that it is also a force of production imbued with particular meanings and materialities. It thus functions as an assembled object in ways that overlap with the doings of a chair. In the context of DMD, the twinned notions of decline and death act as agentic absent-presences that make and unmake person-care objects and subjects of particular types.

Death has a rich and complicated history. While an exploration of this history is beyond the scope of this paper, a couple of remarks are needed before considering death in relation to becoming-michael. The frequent personification of death in literature, religion, and popular culture speaks to its powers of intervention, and its ontological status is an ancient and continuing point of philosophical debate. Deleuze for his part rejected notions that life is oriented towards death, that death does or should mediate how life is lived, or even that death is an endpoint of life (Deleuze, 1988). He saw such formulations as inventions of a territorialised structure that limits possibilities and impedes lines of flight (Baugh, 2000). He nevertheless acknowledged the need to 'keep enough of the organism for it to reform each dawn' i.e. not to deterritorialise too much or risk dying (Deleuze & Guattari, 1987, p. 160). Deleuze's notions of death paralleled his rejection of the static subject contained within a biological body, i.e. becoming cannot accommodate death as endpoint because there is no individual to perish. In defanging death, he called for an open-ended plugging in of desiring machines, forming and reforming assemblages, and achieving intensities.

For our analysis, we similarly avoid anchoring death to essentialised persons while still considering it as a constructed force of production pervading biomedicine, clinical encounters, and the doings of everyday life. In the clinic, decline-towards-death functions as a material-semiotic object that interacts with diagnosis and other forces to territorialise DMD and instigate a host of activities. Dominant notions of death [as well as life] are affective. They do things, make subjects and lives of a certain kind. In the DMD clinic, loss of muscle strength is understood as degeneration and decline; similarly, DMD is positioned as a 'life-limiting' or 'palliative' condition. In coming into relation with DMD, decline thus marks the body as disabled in a negative register. The doings of the clinic, oriented to preserving life and slowing decline, produce and sustain affective spaces of loss, hope, struggle etc. With these ideas in mind, we return to becoming-michael.

Medical research suggests that 29 years is the average life expectancy of DMD (Landfeldt et al., 2020). We use this wording deliberately – DMD lives to be 29, maybe longer. There are new treatments and drugs. Sometimes DMD lives to 40 and even 50 in particular configurations of biology, treatments, resources, motivations. DMD is always becoming-death but also becoming-life. M/michael is implicated in this assemblage of becoming-death/life and its effects in and beyond clinic spaces. Death entangles with becoming-michael, with the family, and with the clinicians. Or instead of 'with' we might say that death makes michael and michael makes death in a unique co-production that vacillates with other forces, bodies, settings. Different material-semiotic objects (michael, death, decline, family, clinic, diagnosis) are enacted, centred, or de-centred, through affective acts of categorisation with a 'looping' effect (Hacking, 2007). DMD is, amongst other things, teen-becoming-death/life with unique properties – a relatively short life trajectory that remains highly uncertain and varies widely. In clinical encounters, uncertainty intersects with hope but also despair, as different affordances create opportunities to enact or block affective flows. Obligatory hope circles into the flow when there is an advance in biomedicine – a new drug, genome editing (Ousterout et al., 2015). Client/son/teen-with-DMD might not die tragically, because new interventions might become available.

Within the biomedical cure-hope assemblage, there is little space for living well in the present or alternative notions of what comprises a good life/time (Gibson, Zitzelsberger, & McKeever, 2009). Becoming-michael's refusals (of employments programs, of the wheelchair) reject the logics of futurity, preservation, and prevention that pervade clinic practices. Safety protocols and employment programs disavow creative possibilities for life in the present, of new ways of being and doing. Biomedicine produces declining-body through quantitative measures, protocols for maintaining the numbers – fixing the body, elevating mood through drugs. Through rehabilitation processes, declining-body is client-with-DMD, the putty for a normalisation project, the making of a life that approximates normal function and independence. Within these configurations, becoming-michael-chair-anime-home-pleasure, to return to our first experiment, is differentially enacted to deterritorialise dying-client. Multiple assemblages co-exist in the micro-politics of care but that does not mean that no-body suffers.

Becoming-death/life raises a consideration of a posthumanist affirmative ethics. Within the spectre of decline, assemblages are enacted, not always experienced as positive but not always conventionally 'tragic' either. Smith (2012) suggests that the fundamental question of a Deleuzian ethics is not '"What *must* I do?" (which is the question of *morality*) but rather "What *can* I do", what am I *capable* of doing (which is the proper question of ethics *without* morality)' (p. 176). Drawing on this ethics, he suggests a set of questions that might inform person-care in our project: 'Given my degree of power, what are my capabilities and capacities? How can I come into active possession of my power? How can I go to the limit of what I can do?' A 'good' or 'healthy' life in such an ethics is open-ended and available to all. This creative expression of life works towards maximising capacities in new, multiple, and different modes, plugging into other assemblages, exploring what can be done. In the clinic, care towards death is always staving-off rather than becoming. Abrams and Adkins (2020) in sketching an affirmative understanding of tragedy suggest that treating decline and disability as an intrusion on life rather than life itself cannot embrace life. Given these notions, how then can person-care reorient to affirming life, desire, power?

If health/life is a process rather than outcome, maximising capabilities invites differential modes of becoming for M/michael. The context of DMD and its relations, where life expectancies are shortened and highly uncertain, affords a line of flight from dominant social and medical life/time temporalities, for becoming-healthy otherwise. M/michael's refusals coalesce opportunities to become-healthy in ways that are not limited to medical goals: maximising potentials to connect with others (humans and things), live well in the present, becoming normal differently, actualising the virtual. Becoming-healthy for M/michael may, for example, include being supported to explore the joys and possibilities of plugging into an anime community, enacting a here-and-now life that departs from the biomedical rendering of the 'deteriorating' body-at-risk. The clinical care encounter could work more deliberately to help coordinate actions and build communities to enable such pursuits. Such efforts include, but do not always or necessarily prioritise, maximising physiological functions or promoting employment/productivity goals along normalised life/time trajectories.

Decentred person-care

Our posthuman experimentations suggest some openings for reimagining persons, care, and thus person-centred care or, as we have suggested, 'person-care'. De-centring signals that person-care is an act of worlding that is always already mediated and re/produced. Becoming makes care and makes persons through a care-full ethics of openness that approaches care as an in-the-moment recognition of productive potentials for doing differently. When care is approached only as a means-to-an-end it continually re/creates the biomedical client-as-lack – a body–object in need of care. In so doing, the binary of patient/carer, the separation of humans and 'context', and the individuation of persons who need to be centred are reasserted. Instead, de-centred person-care is care that explores possibilities: What can this assemblage create or produce that is care-full? That affirms becoming-life? The point is not to ignore the interpersonal, but to highlight that in assemblages of becoming, new ways of being are created that resist reinforcing inequities and anxieties. The emphasis, then, is placed not on 'what can you do for me?' but rather 'what we can create together?' (Fritsch, 2010). How can one act/ think/ feel to affirm life, desire, power? To activate powers of production towards making a life, asking what capabilities and capacities are available, what powers can be mobilised? How can life go to the limits of what it can do?

Elsewhere we have described creative and open clinical processes using the terminology of tinkering (Gibson et al., 2020). Tinkering is emplaced doing, asking: What is going on here? How can the tools at hand be mobilised to make life better? Toro and Martiny (2020) refer to reciprocal 'we-interactions' between professionals, patients, and families as facilitating PCC. We agree but suggest that the 'we' extends beyond the humans in the room and acknowledge all of the material-semiotic forces that conspire to produce person-care. Decentred person-care mobilises forces of production, imagines new assemblages, new doings, and tinkers with the im/possible. Everything is available from office chairs to death in making life. What affirmative machines can be made?

Becoming-michael's refusals could have catalyzed re-fusing, that is a reordering of the territorialised imperatives of safety and normalisation that pervade clinical practices. Something amiss with michael could instigate change, new person-care becomings. How to pivot from becoming-anime affective pleasures to creatively actualise the virtual yet-to-be michaels? What else can be done to enable becoming-michael that cares for and about Michael-client, and about Jee-parent? Refusal is not an end point or something that needs to be 'dealt with' (through 'patient education', cajoling, reasoning) it provides a time-place to stop, swivel, plug in differently. Could the professionals set aside concerns for joint alignment or safety and work with the creativity of body-chair? What capacities coalesce with body-chair; how else could it plug in? Decentred person-care experiments with thinking-as-usual towards re-envisioning differences as potentials rather than deficits. What is blocking desire and how might it be rearranged? What 'ontological styles' can be created that exceed the boundaries of body, chair, and subject? This is not easy or necessarily 'better' but is an available alternative for affirming life. Such approaches bring other forces into the mix, they recognise the driving affects that produce client-with-DMD, recognise what subject positions work to achieve, look for other possibilities to help parent–child affirm life.

The analysis of person-care is not utopian but grounded in reimagining ossified modes of practice in contemporary healthcare environments. Theorising difference through experimentation works to disrupt the entrenched and remake the world, resisting territorialisations of care, and opening new ways of re/forming PCC and health care practices. New understandings of emergent care processes are brought in conversation with existing ways of doing and knowing to generate something new. These analyzable events and assemblages transform the unimaginable into the doable (Ness, 2011) and new ground is gained in making livable worlds.

Coda

Our task was one of problem-producing rather than problem-solving. The latter tends to close off creative modes of thinking. In conceptualising PCC differently, in making new problems that did not previously exist, we worked to expand and transform the limitations of dominant methodologies and epistemological commitments. As a clinician-researcher assemblage, we reflexively sought to discover how our positions, experiences, and commitments informed our analyses and challenged ourselves to sit with discomfort and uncertainty in experimenting with PCC. In these efforts, there are inevitable gaps and interpretations that led us to map assemblages in ways that are always and necessarily partial. An assemblage can have an entry point but never an exit. Indeed, in this particular 'case', questions may be raised about all kinds of 'missing' facts and forces, for example related to other social positions and political realities that enact the subject positions of michael and others. We attend to these ideas with a deep humility, knowing that we saw and attended to some forces and not others, and in this risk contributing to various harms that may not be easily identified or named. These particularities highlight how cases are always partial, and that the sort of analysis we had embarked on opens as many questions and possibilities as it attempts to produce. To this end, we welcome further debate and discussion.

Acknowledgements

The authors would like to thank the following who participated in the original study discussed in the paper: Laura McAdam, Thomas Abrams, Bhavnita Mistry, Jenny Setchell, Patricia Thille, and the study participants. Barbara Gibson was supported by the Bloorview Kids Foundation Chair in Childhood Disability Studies.

Disclosure statement

No potential conflict of interest was reported by the author(s).

ORCID

Barbara E. Gibson http://orcid.org/0000-0003-0429-8679
Joanna K. Fadyl http://orcid.org/0000-0001-7678-9122
Gareth Terry http://orcid.org/0000-0002-6377-6194
Kate Waterworth http://orcid.org/0000-0002-3777-0688
Donya Mosleh http://orcid.org/0000-0002-3630-9945
Nicola M. Kayes http://orcid.org/0000-0002-2747-667X

References

Abrams, T., & Adkins, B. (2020). Tragic affirmation: Disability beyond optimism and pessimism. *Journal of Medical Humanities*. Advance online publication. doi:10.1007/s10912-020-09612-y

Abrams, T., & Gibson, B. E. (2017). Putting Gino's lesson to work: Actor–network theory, enacted humanity, and rehabilitation. *Health: An Interdisciplinary Journal for the Social Study of Health, Illness and Medicine*, *21*(4), 425–440.

Abrams, T., Setchell, J., Thille, P., Mistry, B., & Gibson, B. E. (2019). Affect, intensity, and moral assemblage in rehabilitation practice. *BioSocieties*, *14*(1), 23–45.

Andrews, G. J., & Duff, C. (2019). Matter beginning to matter: On posthumanist understandings of the vital emergence of health. *Social Science & Medicine*, *226*, 123–134.

Barad, K. (2003). Posthumanist performativity: Toward an understanding of how matter comes to matter. *Signs: Journal of Women in Culture and Society*, *28*(3), 801–831.

Baugh, B. (2000). Death and temporality in Deleuze and Derrida. *Angelaki: Journal of Theoretical Humanities*, *5*(2), 73–83.

Blume, S., Galis, V., & Pineda, A. V. (2014). Introduction: STS and disability. *Science, Technology & Human Values*, *39*(1), 98–104.

Braidotti, R. (2013). *The posthuman*. Cambridge, UK: Polity Press.

Braidotti, R. (2019). A theoretical framework for the critical posthumanities. *Theory, Culture & Society*, *36*(6), 31–61.

Buse, C., Martin, D., & Nettleton, S. (2018). Conceptualising 'materialities of care': Making visible mundane material culture in health and social care contexts. *Sociology of Health & Illness*, *40*(2), 243–255.

Callon, M., & Rabeharisoa, V. (2004). Gino's lesson on humanity: Genetics, mutual entanglements and the sociologist's role. *Economy and Society*, *33*(1), 1–27.

Carlson, D. L., Wells, T. C., Mark, L., & Sandoval, J. (2021). Introduction: Working the tensions of the post-qualitative movement in qualitative inquiry. *Qualitative Inquiry*, *27*(2), 151–157.

Deleuze, G. (1978). *Gilles Deleuze, Lecture transcripts on Spinoza's concept of affect*. Lecture, Les Cours Vincennes. https://www.webdeleuze.com/textes/14.

Deleuze, G. (1988). *Spinoza: Practical philosophy*. San Francisco, CA: City Lights Books.

Deleuze, G., & Guattari, F. (1987). *A thousand plateaus: Capitalism and schizophrenia*. Minneapolis, MN: University of Minnesota Press.

Edvardsson, D., & Innes, A. (2010). Measuring person-centered care: A critical comparative review of published tools. *The Gerontologist, 50*(6), 834–846.

Fox, N. J., & Alldred, P. (2017). *Sociology and the new materialism: Theory, research, action.* London, UK: Sage.

Fox, N. J., & Alldred, P. (2018). Mixed methods, materialism and the micropolitics of the research-assemblage. *International Journal of Social Research Methodology, 21*(2), 191–204.

Fritsch, K. (2010). Intimate assemblages: Disability, intercorporeality, and the labour of attendant care. *Critical Disability Discourses, 2.* https://cdd.journals.yorku.ca/index.php/cdd/article/view/23854/28098.

Fullagar, S., O'Brien, W., & Pavlidis, A. (2019). *Feminism and a vital politics of depression and recovery.* Cham, Switzerland: Springer.

Gibson, B. E. (2006). Disability, connectivity and transgressing the autonomous body. *Journal of Medical Humanities, 27*(3), 187–196.

Gibson, B. E. (2014). Parallels and problems of normalization in rehabilitation and universal design: Enabling connectivities. *Disability and Rehabilitation, 36*(16), 1328–1333.

Gibson, B. E., Terry, G., Setchell, J., Bright, F. A., Cummins, C., & Kayes, N. M. (2020). The micro-politics of caring: Tinkering with person-centered rehabilitation. *Disability & Rehabilitation, 42* (11), 1529–1538.

Gibson, B. E., Zitzelsberger, H., & McKeever, P. (2009). 'Futureless persons': Shifting life expectancies and the vicissitudes of progressive illness. *Sociology of Health & Illness, 31*(4), 554–568.

Guastello, S., & Jay, K. (2019). Improving the patient experience through a comprehensive performance framework to evaluate excellence in person-centred care. *BMJ Open Quality, 8*(4), e000737.

Hacking, I. (2007). Kinds of people: Moving targets. In *Proceedings-British academy,* (p. 151). Oxford, UK: Oxford University Press. https://www.thebritishacademy.ac.uk/documents/2043/pba151p285.pdf

Holford, W. D. (2020). The algorithmic workplace and its enactive effect on the future of professions. *Futures, 122.* doi:10.1016/j.futures.2020.102609

Holmes, D., Murray, S. J., Perron, A., & Rail, G. (2006). Deconstructing the evidence-based discourse in health sciences: Truth, power and fascism. *International Journal of Evidence-Based Healthcare, 4*(3), 180–186.

Landfeldt, E., Thompson, R., Sejersen, T., McMillan, H. J., Kirschner, J., & Lochmüller, H. (2020). Life expectancy at birth in Duchenne muscular dystrophy: A systematic review and meta-analysis. *European Journal of Epidemiology, 35*(7), 643–653.

Leder, D. (1990). *The absent body.* Chicago, IL: University of Chicago Press.

Leplege, A., Gzil, F., Cammelli, M., Lefeve, C., Pachoud, B., & Ville, I. (2007). Person-centredness: Conceptual and historical perspectives. *Disability and Rehabilitation, 29*(20–21), 1555–1565.

Massumi, B. (1992). *A user's guide to capitalism and schizophrenia: Deviations from Deleuze and Guattari.* Cambridge, MA: MIT Press.

Mol, A. (2008). *The logic of care: Health and the problem of patient choice.* London, UK: Routledge.

Monforte, J., & Smith, B. (2021). Conventional and postqualitative research: An invitation to dialogue. *Qualitative Inquiry, 27*(6), 650–660.

Moser, I. (2006). Disability and the promises of technology: Technology, subjectivity and embodiment within an order of the normal. *Information, Communication & Society, 9*(3), 373–395.

Ness, S. A. (2011). Bouldering in Yosemite: Emergent signs of place and landscape. *American Anthropologist, 113*(1), 71–87.

Ousterout, D. G., Kabadi, A. M., Thakore, P. I., Majoros, W. H., Reddy, T. E., & Gersbach, C. A. (2015). Multiplex CRISPR/Cas9-based genome editing for correction of dystrophin mutations that cause Duchenne muscular dystrophy. *Nature Communications, 6*(1), 1–13.

Sandelowski, M. (2011). "Casing" the research case study. *Research in Nursing & Health, 34*(2), 153–159.

Saxton, M., Curry, M. A., Powers, L. E., Maley, S., Eckels, K., & Gross, J. (2001). "Bring my scooter so I can leave you" a study of disabled women handling abuse by personal assistance providers. *Violence Against Women, 7*(4), 393–417.

Setchell, J., Thille, P., Abrams, T., McAdam, L. C., Mistry, B., & Gibson, B. E. (2018). Enhancing human aspects of care with young people with muscular dystrophy: Results from a participatory qualitative study with clinicians. *Child: Care, Health and Development*, *44*(2), 269–277.

Shouse, E. (2005). Feeling, emotion, affect. *M/C Journal*, *8*(6). doi:10.5204/mcj.2443

Smith, D. (2012). *Essays on Deleuze*. Edinburgh, UK: Edinburgh University Press.

Smith, D. W. (2020). The Deleuzian revolution: Ten innovations in difference and repetition. *Deleuze and Guattari Studies*, *14*(1), 34–49.

Toro, J., & Martiny, K. (2020). New perspectives on person-centered care: An affordance-based account. *Medicine, Health Care and Philosophy*, *23*, 631–644.

OPEN ACCESS

Materialities of care for older people: caring together/apart in the political economy of caring apparatus

Michela Cozza, Silvia Bruzzone and Lucia Crevani

ABSTRACT

By applying a posthuman perspective to the analysis of care for older people (COP), we analyse the agential cuts (together/apart) enacted by humans (mainly caregivers and older people) and more-than-humans (a camera intra-acting with other objects) whose agential entanglement configures and reconfigures the political economy of the caring apparatus. Our study identifies 'targeting', 'monitoring', and 'aligning' as interrelated caring practices, thus contributing to advance a posthuman understanding of welfare technology, and advancing a critical use of the possibilities enacted by technologies.

Introduction

Care for older people (COP)[1] is, in many countries of the Global North,[2] conceived of as an exclusive human matter. As we witness the increasing use of digital technologies in providing welfare services to older people, such a transformation changes the way we understand COP, and the practices of caring for older people are hence reconstructed. In this paper, we thus propose to mobilise critical posthumanism to account for how an artefact – the night camera (henceforth: camera) – becomes part of and affects COP in a Swedish municipality. This camera is part of a larger infrastructure for remote monitoring of older people at home. The service is owned by the municipality and consists of technological equipment (the core is constituted by the camera linked to a router installed at users' home and interoperating with computers at the municipal operations centre) and a variety of professional caregivers differently involved in assessing the need for the equipment and making it work properly to assure that home care service is delivered to users in compliance with the national law and local (regional and municipal) policies.

Sweden provides a particularly interesting context, since homecare[3] is a welfare benefit to which all citizens are eligible. Due to an ageing population, as well as budget restrictions and a decrease in the professional vocation in home-caring, the so-called 'welfare technologies' (devices used in welfare services) have been increasingly envisioned as the solution. Moreover, the digital transformation has also become a prioritised policy area to re-affirm Sweden as one of the most digitally innovative countries in the world. Municipalities are thus faced with new policies and practices that are expected to satisfy citizens' needs and rights. Despite much attention paid to welfare technologies, their role remains underestimated and unexplored as regards the reconfiguration of existing care practices, policy strategies, and new ethical dilemmas. Controversial issues thus emerge, and decisions made regarding a single device, such as the camera, may contribute to re-arrange COP at large.

Literature discussing the materialities of COP (see below) highlights the active role of objects in care, which we will conceive of as 'more-than-human caregivers'. These studies also provide lenses to analyse caring practices, through the mundane materiality of a more-than-human caregiver such as the camera. Our aim is to explore the possibilities and exclusions produced and reproduced in caring practices when policies of welfare technology and digitalisation lead to the introduction of more-than-human caregivers, in our case the camera. Building on Karen Barad's 'agential realism', we will analyse how the political economy of what we propose as the 'caring apparatus' is articulated through different practices. That is, we will attend to practices emerging in the entanglement of older people, professionals, and technologies (which, together, form the *caring apparatus*), and reproducing specific configurations of care, which in turn differentiates caring for different older people, depending on which interests are included and excluded (*political economy*). This argument is not only theoretical, but even demonstrates the need for posthuman thought to engage with and care for materialities in COP.

Materialities of care for older people

The significance of materialities has attracted increasing attention within the sociology of health and illness, situated within traditions of science and technology studies (STS) and new materialism. We use 'materialities of COP' as a heuristic device (Buse, Martin, & Nettleton, 2018), where mundane materialities act as a lens for studying care practices in welfare technology, that is, the technology used to improve welfare services and make them more efficient (Nordic Centre for Welfare and Social Issues, 2010). Materialities of COP encompasses ideas of both 'materiality' and 'care', which are not univocally defined. Here we focus on materialities not only as physical 'things', but also as networks of socio-material assemblages of people, objects, and technologies (a camera is our focus here) (Fox, 2016; Lovatt, 2018). Therefore, we do not frame materialities as 'merely a backdrop for care interactions, but playing an active role in constituting relations of care' (Buse, Martin & Nettleton, 2018).

Overall, the debate on materialities of COP has received a substantial contribution from a developing interdisciplinary field within the study of ageing, known as 'material gerontology' (e.g. Höppner, 2017; Höppner & Urban, 2018; Wanka & Gallistl, 2018). We situate our contribution to this research as a study of the interrelations between ageing and technology *from an organisational perspective*, a field still highly resistant to posthumanism (Bell, Meriläinen, Taylor, & Tienari, 2020). Studies falling under material gerontology deal, for example, with the meaning of objects for older adults, and older adults' construction of identity, for instance using clothing but also wearable technologies (Cozza, 2021; Long, 2012). Some authors explore the role of objects in the context of care, including homecare (Loe, 2010; Mort, Roberts, & Callén, 2013). In this regard, scholars influenced by STS have analysed the social and societal implications of technologies, with special attention paid to remote monitoring technologies. Among these scholars, some focus on power and aspects of domination, and widely draw from Michel Foucault's work on health, illness, and micropolitics of surveillance (Essén, 2008; Joyce & Loe, 2010; Mort et al., 2013). We acknowledge the role of post-structuralism that Foucault initiated, in examining the micropolitics of health care (Fox, 2016, 2017). However, we also point out that post-structuralism made discourses, text, and textuality the object of study, while the materiality of the body receded beyond the analytical purview of the social scientist. Reacting to the post-structuralist denial of the materiality of the body, a 'material turn' emerged (Wanka & Gallistl, 2018) 'to bring back to discourses on the body (…) the materiality of humans and their material environments under specific conditions' (Höppner, 2017, p. 2). New materialism claims that the capacity for 'agency' – the actions that produce the social world and emerge through relationships – extends beyond human actors to the more-than-humans. For example, Lupton, by drawing on Donna Haraway's work, talks about 'digital data assemblages as companion species that have a life of their own that is beyond our complete control' (2016, p. 3); accordingly, adopting a more-than-human approach 'demands that the human subject is always considered permeable and open to the material world rather than closed-off and contained' (2018, p. 4). From this perspective, the same humanist idea of 'body' is challenged: a body is not something that 'exists' or 'is', but rather 'does' through intra-actions (Fullagar, Rich, Pavlidis, & van Ingen, 2019) – a concept that we explain below.

Therefore, the question 'who acts' – by assuming caring as the action or rather the apparatus of material-discursive practices we focus on – is expanded into the question 'what acts'. This is consistent with a concept of agency as relational, rather than conceived as an a priori and given feature of a human actor. Agency emerges from the interrelations between heterogeneous actors whose assemblage constitutes care practices (Reckwitz, 2012). Given this, the materialities of COP refer to bodies, objects, technological artefacts, possessions, relations, and knowledge, among other things, which are mutually entangled in specific situations. How they are entangled, however, depends on the apparatus and 'agential cuts' considered below.

Caring apparatus

Care is a contested and diverse concept, as pointed out by Mol (2006), who argues for disentangling 'care' from an anthropocentric idea associated with kindness, dedication, and generosity, which are crucial but cast care as opposed to technology. 'Care' is not opposed to, but includes and embodies technology. The technology we refer to 'is not transparent and predictable, but has to be handled with care' (Mol, 2006, p. 6); in turn, care is a practice that 'counts for engagement with "things"' (Puig de la Bellacasa, 2017, p. 29). Such a definition of care as caring resonates with a feminist practice-based approach that frames caring as an emergent process realised by a heterogeneous collective of humans and more-than-humans (Gherardi & Rodeschini, 2016). As Pols writes, 'there is no such thing as technology, but many practices where many different technologies are being used', and 'there is no such thing as care practice, but there are many different care practices' (2017, p. 2).

Especially in the countries of the Global North, COP is increasingly, although not exclusively, treated like any other 'industry'. Older adults are surrounded by a variety of objects (e.g. security alarms, hearing and vision aids, medication reminders, mobile apps), some of which are actively used as deemed to provide care and increase their well-being, while others technologies become more-than-human companions in daily life, and are often chosen for the sake of the family and, above all, for the peace of mind of older people's children. Put differently, ageing is sometimes governed by an open-ended process of caring that involves a team of professionals, devices, bodies, and relevant others (Yakhlef & Essén, 2013); sometimes, ageing is ruled by a unidirectional process according to which older people are passive consumers or customers of products (Peine, Rollwagen, & Neven, 2014) whose being and doing are regulated by the market or, as we posit, by the *political economy* of a caring apparatus. The 'economy' of the apparatus relates to its agency in *producing* and *re-producing* specific configurations of care; the 'political' feature of the apparatus regards the *non-neutrality* of such configurations, which always depends on specific cuts and, ultimately, on particular interests.

Our concept of 'political economy of apparatuses' is based on Karen Barad's (2007, p. 230) agential realism, which has contributed to a new material thinking and has widely influenced the sociomaterial perspective and its notion of constitutive entanglement (Orlikowski, 2007; Orlikowski & Scott, 2008). However, Barad does not apply the concept (i.e. political economy of apparatus) to caring, which is our task here.

The concept of apparatus relies on the neologism 'intra-action' that Barad has formulated in contrast to the standard term 'interaction', which presumes the prior existence of independent entities. Hence, intra-actions include a large material arrangement, a set of material-discursive practices or apparatus, which effects an 'agential cut' between subject and object, between what is excluded and what is included in a specific situation. Agential cuts are, then, non-dualistic practices of differentiation, in sharp contrast to the Cartesian cut that establishes the autonomous, exceptional agency of the humanist subject.

The concept of apparatus in COP allows for analysis of caring practices as enacted by intra-acting human and more-than-human actors, and enables analysis of the multiple ways in which such an apparatus does not simply detect differences already in place (for example, differences between the living conditions of older people, or geographical differences between welfare systems), but rather contributes to the production and reproduction of differences (for example, the abovementioned differences, their enactment by a specific intervention). Therefore, there is no way for the material-discursive caring practices of which an apparatus is made to be 'innocent' (Barad, 1996). '[*C*]*uts* are performative, have materialising effects, which produce entanglements/relations/relationships through and in establishing differences: "cutting together/apart"' (Völker, 2019, p. 91).

'Cutting together/apart', in Barad's work, refers to an apparently paradoxical process that encompasses both entangling (*together*) and differentiating (*apart*), joins and disjoins (Barad, 2013). In other words, and by applying the concept to a caring apparatus, every material-discursive practice inevitably affects in different way different actors, and such consequences materialise as possibilities (for some) and threats (for others).

In this paper, we propose using 'caring together/apart' to refer to specific practices and the cuts enacted by them within the political economy of a caring apparatus. In the case at hand, the political economy of the caring apparatus has not only a theoretical relevance, but also an empirical concreteness, which finds its referents in financial issues and policy matters. Caring practices generate better living possibilities for some older people but, inevitably but not purposefully, include a spectrum of impossibilities for others. By collecting several examples of caring practices under the umbrella-term 'caring together/apart', we want to position the caring apparatus within a politics of possibilities, while acknowledging that the same practice may enact 'im/possibilities'. However, with regard to COP, we propose expanding this original concept by using 'caring together-' to emphasise, on the one hand, what a care practice makes possible and the particular possibilities for intra-acting it opens up, while, on the other hand, we use 'caring -apart' to highlight the constraining nature of specific cuts, that is, what/who is excluded from mattering within the caring apparatus, through that practice.[4] We ground such an articulation of caring apparatus and practices on Barad's concept of agency that opens up to 'possibilities for the iterative reconfiguring of the materialities of human, nonhuman, cyborgian, and other such forms' (2007, pp. 177–178).

The following presentation of COP practices necessarily involves an analysis of the artefacts which are assembled to constitute the caring apparatus we refer to and, in particular, we develop our argument focusing on the case of a camera as a more-than-human caregiver.

Case study method

Our case study relates to the adoption of a camera for older people at home. The context is a Swedish municipality of about 100,000 inhabitants, considered one of Sweden's most innovative cities in welfare technology, thanks to an active network of actors, namely the local university, the regional authority, the municipal government, hospitals, older people associations, and the regional assistive technology centre. The municipality has decided to adopt the camera, deemed to provide 'better', service as people are not disturbed at night compared to when professional caregivers (*Nattpatrullen,* the homecare night patrol) visit them,[5] but also in consideration of the potential savings. Since 2018, 30 cameras have been installed in the municipality (the total number of people having homecare at night is 200 with approximately 400 tasks performed every night).

The empirical material was produced over a period of four years (2016-2020) and results from the collaboration between the local university and public authorities in three national projects on welfare technology for older people. We conducted semi-structured interviews and participatory workshops with older people interested in using welfare technologies (i.e. not only the camera); municipal managers for quality in the care and wellbeing division (*Vård- och Omsorgsförvaltningen*); the digital strategist of the same division responsible for the digital development on care and wellbeing; the project manager of the communication, IT, and digitalisation Unit (*Kommunication, IT och Digitalisering Enhet*); the case officers (*Biståndshandläggare*) who assess the needs of older people and make determinations; and, finally, the head of the night patrol unit, who monitors older people at distance and makes visits as necessary. Along with these interviews, we also interviewed key informants indirectly involved in the implementation of the 'camera strategy', that is, the regional office for the dissemination of knowledge in the health care sector, and the regional assistive technology centre.

We have also conducted ethnographic observations of meetings during the implementation of the camera, and realised further interviews with representatives from companies in the welfare technology market on the occasion of an important annual trade fair in Stockholm, twice attended by two authors (2017, 2018) to collect qualitative data (detailed descriptions of some of these activities can be found Andersson, Cozza, Crevani, & Schunnesson, 2018; Cozza, Crevani, Hallin, & Schaeffer, 2018; Crevani & Cozza, 2018).

In our analysis, we focus on three caring practices (among possible others) embodying the materialisation of the political economy of the caring apparatus in its agential cutting together/apart. Consistent with the posthuman approach, we do not prioritise human voices in presenting data; that is, we do not show our data – for example through quotes – as done in humanist qualitative post-positivist research. Instead, we develop a narrative that allows for appreciation of the complex entanglement between humans and more-than-humans (Fullagar et al., 2019) by acknowledging that devices do not speak, and that what they do can only be observed and spoken about by researchers (Pols, 2012). By narrating, rather than extracting 'evidences' (St. Pierre, 2021), we think through a more-than-human orientation, according to which we foreground the entanglement of heterogeneous actors and, in line with posthuman ethics, we account for the human and more-than-human agency in COP more symmetrically (Fullagar, 2017; Pols, 2015).

Caring practices in a Swedish municipality

In this section, we explore how caring is not the mere result of actions engineered by human subjects, but rather emerges from complex agential intra-actions of multiple material-discursive practices of bodily production. In particular, we identified 'targeting', 'monitoring', and 'aligning' as interrelated caring practices that we unpack and articulate from a posthuman perspective. By these practices, various agential cuts are enacted, which in turn correspond to 'caring together-' and 'caring -apart'.

Targeting

In our reading of the empirical material, targeting emerges as a practice consisting in selecting which older people the caring apparatus should include in (caring together-) or exclude from (caring -apart) welfare care, based on an assessment of their needs. In the following, by recalling the history of the camera and telling it in the form of a story, we point out that care is performed intra-actively by human and more-than-human agents. Among these, the camera is the main (but not exclusive) actor entitled to 'look at' older people remotely, and it partially replaces the human 'colleagues' as the exclusive agents appointed to visit the person at night and ensure their health, safety, and comfort. Such a technology becomes the digital companion of the older person, as well as a more-than-human caregiver, along with the human companions. But let us step back, and examine the origin of this apparatus.

The introduction of this new technological 'member' of the municipal caring staff was based on a debate about which older persons were entitled to remote visits via camera oversight, or, phrased differently, how the camera could meet an older person's needs while supporting the night patrol unit. Indeed, the strangeness of night-time visits to an older person's home, and awakening an older person in the middle of the night, caused distress for both homecare staff and older persons. The camera was thus considered a more respectful and discrete potential agent.

At this point in the story, the camera enters the municipal caring apparatus as an unknown element intra-acting with pre-existing practices aimed at assessing older people's needs first and, as needed, eventually replacing in-person visits with the 'technological gaze' to guarantee peaceful sleep. From a human perspective, this is a tricky question. On the one hand, managers and municipal accountants quickly realised the possible savings that the camera could bring, since time for visits and travel would be reduced. Hence, the possibility of targeting older people in the name of financial issues began materialising in the local caring apparatus.

On the other hand, case officers worried about taking responsibility for finalising the needs assessment by, consciously or not, promoting the camera. Such a decision would meet financial targets and, probably, would please some older people; at the same time, it would cut -apart other older people that, for different reasons, are not considered a proper target and, ultimately, could not benefit from the technological assistance. In short, the human caregivers were torn over having to decide how to distribute homecare by taking into account the budgetary issue that seriously affects services, due to limited human and financial resources. The human caregivers realised that, either way, they would generate a diversification among the older population in terms of access to welfare benefits.

In this process that we, as researchers, have been involved with over a period of years, the camera eventually becomes a legitimised caregiver that human caregivers are appointed to include in the home care service package, once an assessment procedure has ascertained its relevance for an individual. From this point of view, the camera becomes both a possibility for some (caring together-) and an exclusion for others (caring -apart), depending on the assessment and consequential targeting. The camera is the first alternative to consider, and only when such a set-up would not work should an in-person visit be considered. This feature of the caring apparatus is also the result of politicians pushing for a quick implementation of this specific technology in the municipality, as a sign of modernity. Despite the fact that the older person's wishes still seem to come first, case officers are supposed to educate older people about how the technology works, and its benefits, something that makes many case officers, who are often ignorant of the device's technical features and wary of seeming pushy, feel uncomfortable. In this regard, professionals involved in the implementation also contribute to further 'cut' the caring process, by constructing a stricter definition of 'need' for the camera in order to accurately targeting the 'right' older people, i.e. those who want it and may become 'allies' in promoting the camera. Municipal accountants even suggest that gathering older people in 'batches', to systematise the implementation of as many cameras as possible at the same time.

The controversial nature of such a caring apparatus is voiced by both case officers and homecare personnel, whose professional ethos frames care as something that everyone has equal right to, whenever necessary, and independent of where one lives, or what public servant provides help from the municipality. This is why, as the camera is implemented, case officers become the bottlenecks in increasing the number of cameras or, in other words, are perceived as antagonists of their technological colleagues.

In our story, as time goes by, new decisions are made. The homecare personnel start installing the camera by themselves, instead of having the camera suppliers doing that, since the most important thing is to place it properly and to interact with the older person while doing that. This new practice also allows homecare personnel to become familiar with the camera, whose adoption and installation they become responsible for, in conversation with older people. This attention for older people is a caring together- practice that, however, rests on a previous process of targeting that cut -apart a number of potential users.

Such a step in the story of the camera leads the caring apparatus to eventually include a human/more-than-human scenario, which combines the physical visits of human caregivers with technological intervention via the camera. Through intra-actions, humans and more-than-humans on the one hand cuts down the expected savings but, on the other hand, respects homecare professionals' ethos as well as gets the gratitude of those older people who feel safer and more secure with such a caring apparatus.

In sum, our data analysis shows that the caring apparatus works through a practice of targeting older people as potential users of the camera. Such a practice makes the apparatus highly controversial, in the way that it creates possibilities for some older people (caring together-) and excludes others (caring -apart) depending on the assessment of their needs. In other words, the targeting produces a diversification within the older population in terms of access to welfare benefits.

Monitoring

Relying on our analysis, we define monitoring as the caring apparatus keeping track of the person it cares for. In this regard, the camera becomes the more-than-human actor entitled to perform such a caring practice, and which enacts caring together- or caring -apart cuts. It is noteworthy that for the camera to perform caring, the case officer and the older person must agree on how often the camera should be active each night (typically a few times) and what the (human) homecare worker should do if the older person is not in the expected place,[6] or if the technology stops working. Practices enacted may include checking again after a few minutes, calling the older person on the phone, and sending night patrol to the old person's home. That said, we can return to the story of the camera and certain missing pieces.

The camera must be ordered from a private supplier which, initially, was also responsible for installing it. However, as mentioned earlier, homecare workers took over this task, since they are more familiar with the older people's routines, preferences, and lifestyles. This caring attention (caring together-) increases older people's trust in the camera and in the homecare apparatus overall. The camera monitors the user through infrared light,[7] so that is 'only' the shape of the body that can be seen remotely on the night patrol's screen. Infrareds are considered more discreet (care together-) than normal cameras used in the pilot study (Figure 1).

A light signal informs older people that the more-than-human caregiver (i.e. the camera) and the human caregivers at distance, are intra-actively monitoring the

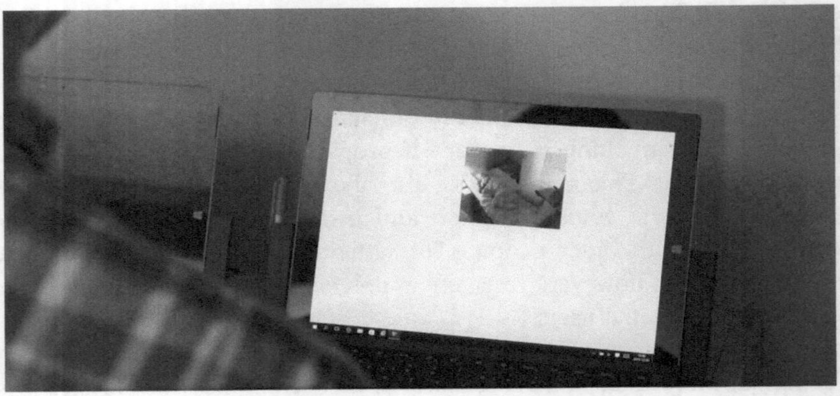

Figure 1. An operator remotely monitors an older person sleeping at home by using a non-infrared camera, during the pilot study.

person at home. The significance of this little light is shown by a story collected in our research, in which a woman waits in her bed for the light to turn on, then waves at the camera. The camera intra-acts with the older person, with the human caregivers in a large open-plan office in the city centre, and also with screens that nevertheless are entangled with the wider sociomaterial caring apparatus.

All tasks performed in relation to one care recipient, as well as all communication with other professionals about a specific user, are logged into an IT application installed on iPads. In June 2019, the municipality had approximately 30 cameras installed and made approximately 70 'looks' during one night-shift, 8:30 pm to 7:00 am. In the case of older people afraid of falling out of bed, checking in during the night via the camera was deemed sufficient to guarantee peace of mind and good sleep. In contrast, people living with dementia must be comforted, reminded that it is night time, and that they should sleep, which means check-ins via the camera are complemented with in-person visits. Both practices are forms of caring together-, that is, forms of caring for differences among users.

The 'collaboration' with the camera implies that night patrols gradually learn how to read what they see on the screen: the 'language' of the technology must be learned, in order to act professionally. Night patrols know which users are usually up at night, and whether they should worry or not when the older person is not in bed, for instance. As they are emotionally invested in the older people, they also worry about the uncertainty generated by the introduction of a more-than-human colleague: What happens if the technology fails? What happens if a member of the night patrol unit falls ill, since only a few are specialised in this service?

Similarly, neither the professionals nor the users accept the relationship with the camera light-heartedly. On the contrary, it instils a sense of insecurity. Some users perceive the monitoring as a form of surveillance, and not by chance, since this is the market area from which the camera comes. As the head of the night patrol unit explained, he 'met' this camera at an exhibition of technologies for surveillance and security. Professionals assuage such concerns by educating users about how the camera monitors them, and that it is activated only for a few seconds at a pre-determined and agreed upon time. In this way, hopefully with time the user forgets about the camera and stops worrying, allowing caring together- to mitigate the effects of caring -apart.

In short, by analysing the practice of monitoring, we can see that the caring apparatus actualises the effects of the practice of targeting while generating new cuts. Monitoring becomes, in other words, a practice of tracking the older people that the apparatus has deemed entitled to a camera. The collaboration with the more-than-human caregiver causes both a sense of insecurity associated with the fear of surveilling and being surveilled (caring -apart), as well as focusing special attention on the differences among users seen through it (caring together-).

Aligning

Our analysis, finally, leads us to the conclusion that aligning is about re-arrangements in the caring apparatus that make professional practices, older people practices, the camera and other materialities converge and work together to produce care. Care offered by the municipality is regulated by specific laws, both concerning social services, which constitute a right for citizens granted through public authority decisions, and by the handling of personal data in different intra-actions involving IT applications. The caring apparatus is a sociomaterial assemblage of heterogeneous actors that work sometimes in parallel, sometimes together: among the human caregivers, these include case officers, homecare personnel, and nurses, but also IT specialists, accountants, communication officers, and legal officers. For this reason, a working group is established in order to coordinate actions and to map where the effects of specific decisions (i.e. cuts) appear. All these different actors must deal with, at a certain point, one more-than-human caregiver, the camera. However, it is worth noting that the camera was not introduced suddenly, but gradually.

Before municipality-wide implementation could be carried out, a pilot was deemed necessary (Figure 1). Technical solutions deemed successful in one municipality cannot be automatically adopted by another municipality, given, for instance, infrastructural differences in internet access or secure data transmission, or varying distances between the homes of older people. This is a matter of caring together-, because the cut is not accomplished regardless of the local character of the caring apparatus, and contextual characteristics can make big differences in determining which solution to adopt.

At the same time, as new roles are needed to face the increasing sociomaterial complexity of the caring apparatus, new routines within and between administrative divisions, and new ways of communicating and intra-acting with the older people, have to be developed. This takes time, and a number of unexpected issues may emerge during the implementation process, including technology failures.

Once the camera is in use, regardless of the type (infrared or otherwise), night patrols are focused on caring together-, that is, securing the safety of the older person. In this regard, one of the most discussed issues concerns the older person's personal integrity. Such a concern is due to the fact that camera suppliers are unused to working with municipalities on health care matters, but work rather with the private sector, where cameras are used for the surveillance of places, rather than humans. Hence, for the camera to become part of the caring apparatus, the organisational practices of the IT system supplier and at the municipality must adjust to each other, and the supplier's needs must be aligned with the municipality's, in order to exchange information about the older people. Interoperability requires some bricolage, such as use of an application on workers' mobile phones to achieve a two-factor log-in procedure.

More problematic is the lack of a secure system for transferring data about the older person (i.e. the user) from the municipality to the supplier: there is no guarantee that the transmission from the camera is not hacked. To continue with our story, it was thus decided to use pseudonyms, in the form of a combination of letters and numbers, in the system. This was a form of caring together-, to safeguard the older person and mitigate the effects of the technological cut in the caring apparatus. Hence, rather than a name, the camera supplier learns that, for example, 'CV3' needs a camera, and that a camera is installed at CV3, and the information system informs human camera monitors that CV3 needs three check-ins per night. In this scenario, a hacker would be unable to learn the identity of the older person.

Despite its efforts to ensure personal integrity, this technical solution creates another worry, as a legal advisor points, regarding the liability of the municipality. Using a pseudonym could in fact increase the risk of providing the wrong service to an older person, which would have legal consequences. Indeed, the wrong sequence of letters and numbers could be typed into the system, when registering a user, and this error could escape notice, since it is more difficult to remember a pseudonym than a real name. Hence, guaranteeing personal integrity comes at the cost of appropriateness of service: caring together- may become caring -apart.

An overarching question regards who is to own, be responsible for, and maintain the IT application connected to the camera: the night patrol (who is knowledgeable and engaged) or the IT administrators (who have no time, and no first-hand knowledge of the context of use)? Given that the camera can also 'take care of' younger people with cognitive deficiencies, eventually, the long-term ownership is given to the IT unit that is neither area nor age specific. Until this department takes over, the night patrol is responsible for managing the camera.

To conclude, based on our analysis, the practice of aligning – which is effectively connected with targeting and monitoring – qualifies as a working apparatus through processes of convergence between professionals involved in caring practices and making information systems interoperate. When it comes to aligning people, objects, and technologies to deliver homecare, questions regarding personal integrity and organisational liability arise. Mutual adaptations and coordination are enacted, in order to provide a better service (caring together-), but the appropriateness of the service may be threatened by the same solutions developed to account for the older users (caring -apart).

Postscript on the political economy of the caring apparatus

Despite the increasing push towards the digitalisation of the caring sector, there is still a limited understanding of the role of technologies in reconfiguring care practices. Our claim builds on a criticism of the still-dominant anthropocentric approach to caring, which disregards that care is more and more about a matter of the entanglement of different materialities.

Our aim was to apply a posthuman perspective to explore the role of a device for night monitoring of COP in a municipality in Sweden. Based on Karen Barad's agential realism

(2007), and by acknowledging the contributions of other (feminist) scholars contributing a relational understanding of care practices (Lupton, 2016, 2018; Mol, 2006; Pols, 2012, 2015, 2017), we proposed to investigate the political economy of the caring apparatus which is an assemblage of material practices producing and re-producing specific configurations of care that stem from specific political and ethical choices. These decisions create certain possibilities but also generate forms of exclusion (caring together/apart). Consequences of any kind are inevitable and not limited to the implementation of a specific device like the camera. Since 'we' – humans – live in technology-saturated environments, the effects of human-more-than-human assemblages are more pronounced than ever, and raise questions, not least ethical, about what such entanglements bring with them (Lupton, 2016).

In particular, by empirically studying the introduction and use of a camera for older people at home, we have identified three main caring practices – targeting, monitoring, and aligning – as cutting care together and apart. This posthuman take extends previous literature on care practices, particularly for older people, and their relational analysis. While narratively presenting the three caring practices, we emphasise how the professional caregivers' perspective (including the camera as the main more-than-human caregiver) and older people as users emerge from intra-actions. Also, we account for the humans-more-than-humans entanglement as such by developing a posthuman ethical reasoning on caring together/apart and the im/possibilities generated by these practices. In this regard, our ethical approach is aligned with Barad's model of an 'ethics of entanglement' that is aimed at underlying the intra-activity between the world and its human and non-human subjects, and accounting for the consequences of the agential cuts that these subjects enact intra-actively.

What emerges from our study is the controversial nature of the caring apparatus, starting from the question of who the target user should be (*targeting*). As we have shown, the fact of proposing the camera as first choice to all people entitled to have night assistance is experienced as a dilemma for the case officers, whose professional ethos is built on human contact and prevents them from dealing with and promoting technical equipment. This translates into a diversified offering of service, which includes some users and exclude others depending on the case officer who assesses their needs. This process also affects the way in which the actual *monitoring* by the camera is perceived by those who receive the monitoring service: for some, this technological device provides a beneficial sense of security, while for others it is a form of surveillance and control. Lastly, critical issue of personal integrity and organisational liability emerge from *aligning* people, objects, and technologies to deliver homecare, whereby the same solutions may improve the service while also creating new vulnerabilities.

The adoption of the camera reconfigures the 'service'. Various intra-actions generate a different caring apparatus that includes the artefact and human professional caregivers. The specific cuts enacted by these intra-actions show the extent to which the entry of the more-than-human caregiver into the caring apparatus also reconfigures the expectations and needs of humans, both older people and professionals.

The camera is an example of welfare technology that works with humans and, in so doing, constantly 'kicks back' (Barad, 1998) and reclaims its role in the caring apparatus. Acknowledging its agency is not a form of technological determinism. Rather, this acknowledgement entails a reassessment of the working of all actors in their multiple sociomaterial entanglements. Traditional practices of collaboration, coordination, and mutual adaptation between human actors have to be reconfigured in light of the agency of more-than-human co-workers that co-configure the caring apparatus. A posthuman perspective provides us with analytical tools to analyse such a complexity, by accounting for its multiple human and more-than-human agents.

Notes

1. This construct ('care *for* older people') does not imply the passivity of older people as recipients of care, but is formulated to emphasise the socio-institutional regime that regulates welfare services in the research context of this article.
2. 'Global North' is generally understood to refer to countries in Europe and North America, as well as Japan and Australia, characterised by economic and technological growth and an ageing population, among other features.
3. 'Homecare' is health care or supportive care provided by professional caregivers in the individual home where the (older) person lives, as opposed to care provided in group accommodations, like clinics or nursing homes.
4. In using 'caring together-' and 'caring -apart' we keep the hyphen directly attached to the terms that Barad (2013) uses in a joint form, to stay true to the original sense of 'dis-jointness', discontinuity and continuity, separation and entanglement, and the intra-relationships between practices that are interrelated. We are aware of the potential limits of our theoretical stretching, which however is not meant to dichotomise caring practices, rather to ease the understanding of specific aspects that we want to point out.
5. When an older person gets access to the homecare service associated with the camera, he or she also provides keys to municipal homecare staff – or night patrol – permitting homecare staff to enter as necessary and, in particular, to conduct systematic nighttime checks to ensure the older person's wellbeing (the equipment, homecare staff, and the sociotechnical process involved have been thoroughly described in Cozza, 2018).
6. Usually the camera is installed in the bedroom.
7. During the pilot study, the camera in use was not infrared (Figure 1).

Disclosure statement

No potential conflict of interest was reported by the author(s).

Funding

This work was supported by Vinnova, under Grant *SInS-Att utveckla förmågan att driva social innovation genom teknik i samverkan* [2016-03170]; under Grant *IVRIS-Att Introducera Välfärdsteknik genom Realisering av Innovationsförmåga i Samverkan* [2018-02955]; and by SKL via Nationella hjälpmedelschefs nätverket, Samhällskontraktet och Regionförbundet Sörmaland och Rekarne Sparbanksstiftelse, under Grant *HV3D-Hjälpmedel och välfärdsteknik i tre dimensioner: ekonomi, organisation och individuella värden* [2016-2405].

ORCID

Michela Cozza http://orcid.org/0000-0002-6998-5034
Silvia Bruzzone http://orcid.org/0000-0003-2130-2158
Lucia Crevani http://orcid.org/0000-0003-2294-7898

References

Andersson, C., Cozza, M., Crevani, L., & Schunnesson, J. (2018, June 4–8). *Infrastructuring for remote night monitoring: Frictions in striving for transparency when digitalising care service.* Proceeding of the 16th European Conference on computer-supported cooperative work, Nancy, France.

Barad, K. (1996). Meeting the Universe Halfway: realism and social constructivism without contradiction. In L. H. Nelson & J. Nelson (Eds.), *Feminism, science, and the philosophy of science* (pp. 161–194). Dordrecht: Springer.

Barad, K. (1998). Getting real: Technoscientific practices and the materialization of reality. *Differences: A Journal of Feminist Cultural Studies, 10*(2), 87–128. https://link.gale.com/apps/doc/A54772266/LitRC?u=malard&sid=LitRC&xid=f4fb64ca

Barad, K. (2007). *Meeting the Universe Halfway: Quantum physic and the entanglement of matter and meaning.* Durham: Duke University Press.

Barad, K. (2013). Ma(r)king time: Material entanglements and re-memberings: Cutting together-apart. In P. R. Carlile, D. Nicolini, A. Langley, & H. Tsoukas (Eds.), *How matter matters. Objects, artifacts, and materiality in organization studies* (pp. 16–31). Oxford: Oxford University Press.

Bell, E., Meriläinen, S., Taylor, S., & Tienari, J. (2020). Dangerous knowledge: The political, personal, and epistemological promise of feminist research in management and organization studies. *International Journal of Management Reviews, 22*(2), 177–192. doi:10.1111/ijmr.12221

Buse, C., Martin, D., & Nettleton, S. (2018). Conceptualising 'materialities of care': Making visible mundane material culture in health and social care contexts. *Sociology of Health & Illness, 40*(2), 243–255. doi:10.1111/1467-9566.12663

Cozza, M. (2018). Interoperability and convergence for welfare technology. In J. Zhou & G. Salvendy (Eds.), *Human aspects of IT for the aged population. Applications in health, assistance, and entertainment.* ITAP 2018. Lecture Notes in Computer Science (Vol. 10927, pp. 13–24). Cham: Springer.

Cozza, M. (2021). Elderliness. The agential inseparability of ageing and assistive technologies. In A. Peine, B. Marshall, W. Martin, & L. Neven (Eds.), *Socio-gerontechnology – interdisciplinary critical studies of ageing and technology* (pp. 70–84). Abingdon, New York: Routledge.

Cozza, M., Crevani, L., Hallin, A., & Schaeffer, J. (2018). Future ageing: Welfare technology practices for our future older selves. *Futures. The Journal of Policy, Planning and Futures Studies, 109*, 117–129. doi:10.1016/j.futures.2018.03.011

Crevani, L., & Cozza, M. (2018). Complementary representational practices for articulating matters of concern. In *Proceedings of the 5th Participatory Innovation Conference 2018* (pp. 270–277). Eskilstuna. http://pin-c.sdu.dk/2018.html

Essén, A. (2008). The two facets of electronic care surveillance: An exploration of the views of older people who live with monitoring devices. *Social Science & Medicine, 67*, 128–136. doi:10.1016/j.socscimed.2008.03.005

Fox, N. J. (2016). Health sociology from post-structuralism to the new materialisms. *Health: An Interdisciplinary Journal for the Social Study of Health, Illness and Medicine, 20*(1), 62–74. doi:10.1177/1363459315615393

Fox, N. J. (2017). Personal health technologies, micropolitics and resistance: A new materialist analysis. *Health: An Interdisciplinary Journal for the Social Study of Health, Illness and Medicine, 21*(2), 136–153. doi:10.1177/1363459315590248

Fullagar, S. (2017). Post-qualitative inquiry and the new materialist turn: Implications for sport, health and physical culture research. *Qualitative Research in Sport, Exercise and Health, 9*(2), 247–257. doi:10.1080/2159676X.2016.1273896

Fullagar, S., Rich, E., Pavlidis, A., & van Ingen, C. (2019). Feminist knowledges as interventions in physical cultures. *Leisure Sciences, 41*(1-2), 1–16. doi:10.1080/01490400.2018.1551163

Gherardi, S., & Rodeschini, G. (2016). Caring as a collective knowledgeable doing: About concern and being concerned. *Management Learning, 47*(3), 266–284. doi:10.1177/1363459315610030

Höppner, G. (2017). Rethinking socialization research through the lens of new materialism. *Frontiers in Sociology, 2*(13), 1–9. doi:103389/fsoc.2017.00013

Höppner, G., & Urban, M. (2018). Where and how do aging processes take place in everyday life? Answers from a new materialist perspective. *Frontiers in Sociology*, *3*(7), 1–9. doi:10.3389/fsoc.2018.00007

Joyce, K., & Loe, M. (2010). A sociological approach to ageing, technology and health. *Sociology of Health and Illness*, *32*(2), 171–180. doi:10.1111/j.1467-9566.2009.01219.x

Loe, M. (2010). Doing it my way: Old women, technology and wellbeing. *Sociology of Health and Illness*, *32*(2), 319–334. doi:10.1111/j.1467-9566.2009.01220.x

Long, S. O. (2012). Bodies, technologies, and aging in Japan: Thinking about old people and their silver products. *Journal of Cross-Cultural Gerontology*, *27*, 119–137. doi:10.1007/s10823-012-9164-3

Lovatt, M. (2018). Becoming at home in residential care for older people: A material culture perspective. *Sociology of Health & Illness*, *40*(2), 366–378. doi:10.1111/1467-9566.12568

Lupton, D. (2016, January–June). Digital companion species and eating data: Implications for theorising digital data-human assemblages. *Big Data & Society*, 1–5. doi:10.1177/2053951715619947

Lupton, D. (2018, July–December). How do data come to matter? Living and becoming with personal data. *Big Data & Society*, 1–11. doi:10.1177/2053951718786314

Mol, A. (2006). *The logic of care. Health and the problem of patient choice*. London: Routledge.

Mort, M., Roberts, C., & Callén, B. (2013). Ageing with telecare: Care or coercion in austerity? *Sociology of Health & Illness*, *35*(6), 799–812. doi:10.1111/j.1467-9566.2012.01530.x

Nordic Centre for Welfare and Social Issues. (2010). *Welfare technology – tool box for implementation*. Stokholm: Nordens välfärdscenter.

Orlikowski, W. (2007). Sociomaterial practices: Exploring technology at work. *Organization Studies*, *28*(9), 1435–1448. doi:10.1177/0170840607081138

Orlikowski, W. J., & Scott, S. V. (2008). 10 sociomateriality: Challenging the separation of technology, work and organization. *The Academy of Management Annals*, *2*(1), 433–474. doi:10.1080/19416520802211644

Peine, A., Rollwagen, I., & Neven, L. (2014). The rise of the "innosumer" – rethinking older technology users. *Technological Forecasting & Social Change*, *82*, 199–214. doi:10.1016/j.techfore.2013.06.013

Pols, J. (2012). *Care at a distance*. Amsterdam: Amsterdam University Press.

Pols, J. (2015). Toward an empirical ethics in care: Relations with technologies in health care. *Medicine, Health Care and Philosophy*, *18*, 81–90. doi:10.1007/s11019-014-9582-9

Pols, J. (2017). Good relations with technology: Empirical ethics and aesthetics in case. *Nursing Philosophy*, *18*(1), 1–7. doi:10.1111/nup.12154

Puig de la Bellacasa, M. (2017). *Matters of care. Speculative ethics in more than human wolds*. Minneapolis: University of Minnesota Press.

Reckwitz, A. (2012). Affective spaces: A praxeological outlook. *Rethinking History*, *16*(2), 241–258. doi:10.1080/13642529.2012.681193

St. Pierre, E. A. (2021). Post qualitative inquiry, the refusal of method, and the risk of the new. *Qualitative Inquiry*, *27*(1), 3–9. doi:10.1177/1077800419863005

Völker, S. (2019). "Cutting together/apart" – impulses from Karen Barad's feminist materialism for a relational sociology. In U. Tikvah Kissmann & J. van Loon (Eds.), *Discussing new materialism. Methodological implications for the study of materialities* (pp. 87–106). Wiesbaden: Springer.

Wanka, A., & Gallistl, V. (2018). Doing age in a digitized world – a material praxeology of aging with technology. *Frontiers in Sociology*, *3*(6), 1–16. doi:10.3389/fsoc.2018.00006

Yakhlef, A., & Essén, A. (2013). Practice innovation as bodily skills: The example of elderly home care service delivery. *Organization*, *20*(6), 881–903. doi:10.1177/1350508412458535

Afflexivity in post-qualitative inquiry: prioritising affect and reflexivity in the evaluation of a health information website

Jenny Setchell, Rebecca Olson, Merrill Turpin, Nathalia Costa, Tim Barlott, Kate O'Halloran, Britta Wigginton and Paul Hodges

ABSTRACT

Increasingly, people turn to online sources for health information, creating human-non-human relationalities. Health websites are considered accessible in scope and convenience but can have limited capacity to accommodate complexities. There are concerns about who gets to 'assemble' with these resources, and who is excluded. Guided by Ahmed's socio-political theories of emotions, we questioned our feelings as we intra-acted with a consumer information website about back pain (MyBackPain). This encouraged us to approach resource evaluation in a way that alters conventional rational/cognitive judgement processes. Our inquiry was 'supra-disciplinary' involving public health, sociology, allied health and consumer collaborators. Specifically, we considered *relationality* – the feelings circulating between bodies/objects and implicated in MyBackPain's affective practices; *impressions* – the marks, images or beliefs MyBackPain makes on bodies/objects; and *directionality* – how these intra-actions pushed in some directions and away from others. Although Ahmed would likely not consider herself 'post-humanist', we argue that her socio-political theories of how objects and emotions entangle are of great interest to furthering critical post-human understandings of health. Rather than threatening decision-making, we suggest that feelings (and their affects) are central to it. The article demonstrates the productive potential of critical post-human inquiry in identifying/countering 'othering' possibilities, and catalysing a 'nomadic shift' towards new human-non-human formations.

Introductions: afflexing online health education

Increasingly, people around the globe are turning to online sources for health information (Wang, Shi, & Kong, 2020). Online resources have potential as accessible sources of information and support for people with health conditions, such as lower back pain (LBP). People with LBP consistently report a desire for information about their condition (Brown, 2004; Laerum, Indahl, & Skouen, 2006) and online resources are likely to be valued for their capacity to provide specific information in varied formats. However, LBP websites are consistently rated as 'poor' in overall quality (Butler & Foster, 2003; Hendrick et al., 2012) and do not meet needs of individuals with the condition (Costa, Nielsen, Jull, Claus, & Hodges, 2020).

This empirical and applied article uses post-qualitative inquiry to consider possibilities for crafting health information that is simultaneously 'scientifically rigorous' and avoidant of associated pitfalls such as reduced consideration of complexity. Post-qualitative inquiry is a relatively new approach to research that avoids following rigid research 'structures' such as methodologies/methods and eschews disciplinary boundaries (St. Pierre, 2021). Rather than using predetermined methods, we prioritise theory in considering how to differently create and evaluate health information.

In alignment with post-qualitative inquiry's avoidance of disciplinary constraints, we take a 'supra-disciplinary' approach (described below), bringing into conversation critical affect and emotions theory, technology and post-positivist evidence-based research translation. We use these seemingly disparate elements to analyse and evaluate one case study: a large online health resource designed for people with LBP. To describe this practice, we coin the term 'afflexivity': a process of intentionally reflexively foregrounding affect and emotion in a post-human intra-action with technology where the 'lively' nature of technology (Lupton, 2020) is also considered productive. By exploring afflexivity as an approach to 'evaluating' resources, we offer a different way to enact appraisal, which is conventionally based on 'rational' cognitive (human) processes.

The 'reflexivity' in our approach warrants further explanation. In social science methodology, reflexivity is a practice of knowing 'the world better … as one knows oneself better' (Bourdieu, 2003, p. 289): going beyond interpretation to explicitly examine researchers' thoughts and experiences. Post-humanist scholars such as Barad (2007) and Haraway (1988) have questioned the utility of this understanding of reflexivity as they argue that it comes from the illusionary essentialised 'fixed' position of a person's rationality. Instead, these scholars argue for the use of the concept of diffraction, involving two or more human or non-human entities affecting each other from unfixed positions. However, we argue that concepts such as researcher reflexivity, particularly *critical* reflexivity, do not only occur at an individual level; they also involve efforts to consider multiple shifting positions, particularly when bringing into intra-action multiple disciplinary approaches, and when they involve considerations of the 'collective scientific unconscious embedded in intellectual practices' (Maton, 2003, p. 58). In health pedagogy, reflexivity is discussed as a process of examining not just one's own assumptions but also disciplinary or institutional 'beliefs, values, social and systemic structures' (Kinsella, Caty, Ng, & Jenkins, 2012. NB: these authors use a synonymous term for the concept of reflexivity, namely 'critical reflection'). For this paper, our focus is on the affective, embodied and relational effects of health information. This *afflexive* reconsideration provides suggestions for how to differently re-present health resources.

In the critical post-humanities there is arguably increasing attention to assembling the 'flattened ontology' of post-humanism with the radical ethical insights gained through structuralist and post-structuralist reflexivity. Braidotti (2018) posits that this type of supra-disciplinary nature characterises the emerging field of the critical post-humanities. Supra-disciplinarity is not (only) about blurring disciplinary boundaries but also about the processes through which knowledge claims get produced:

> The point of encounter or assemblage of the critical posthumanities acknowledges the porous nature not only of their institutional boundaries but also of their epistemic core, which gets redefined in terms of relational capacity. (p. 44)

Thus, Braidotti argues, what underpins supra-disciplinary research endeavours is relationality as opposed to either a desire for rigid disciplinary boundaries or opposition to them: 'The driving force for knowledge production is therefore not the quest for disciplinary purity, or the inspirational force of radical dissent, but rather the modes of relation these discourses are able and willing to open up to' (Braidotti, 2018, p. 44). Supra-disciplinary work differs from transdisciplinary work in that the disciplines intra-act. Disciplines are not untouched by their assemblage – they affect each other. In this endeavour, we use a 'supra-disciplinary sensibility' to move towards new approaches.

Our case study examines 'MyBackPain' (Arthritis Australia, 2018), an online resource developed by two of the authors (Jenny Setchell and Paul Hodges) in collaboration with the Cochrane Back and Neck Review Group (an international organisation that produces systematic reviews of health research) and Arthritis Australia (a large national consumer-focussed organisation). Paul was the senior researcher with overarching responsibility for the website including procuring project funding and establishing industry and expert collaborations. Jenny was a research fellow employed to work with the collaborators and website developers, to enact the consultation with industry and consumers, and to populate and edit the developing website using its content management system. Development of the website involved extensive consultation with people living with LBP, clinicians and researchers (Hodges, Setchell, & Nielsen, 2020). Considered a large work of 'research translation', MyBackPain systematically incorporates the review and interpretation of studies on over 80 types of treatments and management strategies for LBP (Arthritis Australia, 2018). The site embodies contemporary post-positivist and clinical understandings of musculoskeletal pain in its key messages: enhancing consumer confidence in self-management and treatment decision-making; encouraging individuals to undertake behaviours that reduce the burden of pain, particularly physical activity; and emphasising reassurance and de-medicalisation of pain (Setchell, Turpin, Costa, & Hodges, 2020).

Positivism is a philosophy of knowledge founded on the assumption that we have access to a concrete reality if we ask the right questions and use 'rigorous' methods (Crotty, 1998; Lincoln, Lynham, & Guba, 2013). *Post*-positivism is a slight relativist shift towards a recognition of a need for some contextualisation of these positivist understandings (Gough & McFadden, 2013; Packer, 2011). Positivism and post-positivism contrast with other approaches to understanding/doing healthcare which, for example, hold that knowledge is always contextual with no singular knowable reality (relativism: Crotty, 1998; Lincoln et al., 2013), or understand reality as in constant flux with boundaries of anything only ever imposed (and thus affected) by who/whatever is observing it (post humanism: Barad, 2007; Deleuze & Guattari, 1987). Post-positivism is the dominant epistemology underpinning health in contemporary Western contexts (Eakin, 2016), including the MyBackPain website (Arthritis Australia, 2018).

The MyBackPain website content is supported by an extensive body of (post-positivist) literature. In this article, we consider potential unintended effects of this type of 'evidence-based' online health information by analysing MyBackPain as a case study. We use socio-political and (new) material conceptualisations of emotion and affect to enact an evaluative process of afflexivity (defined above), prioritising examination of emotions implicit in the website and our interactions with it. Specifically, we draw on theories of affect and emotions in social life from Ahmed (2014) in our evaluative analysis. Although Ahmed would likely not consider herself 'post-humanist', we argue that her socio-political theories of how objects and emotions entangle are of great interest to furthering critical post-human understandings of health. In what follows, we outline some of the key Ahmedian concepts that we will employ, before explaining our post-qualitative approach.

Following Deleuze (1988), many distinguish between affect and emotion. Affect is conceptualised as pre-personal, non-conscious, but embodied and emerging sensations, implicated in shared experiences that sensorially call people to attention and action (Iedema & Carroll, 2015; Massumi, 2002). Deleuze (1988, p. 123) emphasises the tension between objects and objects, objects and humans, and the individual and society in his discussion of affect: 'a body affects all other bodies, or is affected by other bodies; it is this capacity for affecting and being affected that also defines a body in its individuality.' Emotions are understood to be culturally-determined labels that individuals consciously give their internal feeling states (Olson, McKenzie, & Patulny, 2017; Turner & Stets, 2006). Some argue that the distinction between affect and emotion is exaggerated and perpetuates a bifurcated understanding of emotions as internal, cognitive and cultural, and affect as material and relational (Cromby & Willis, 2016; Leys, 2017). Aligned with these critiques, we follow Ahmed (2014) in conceptualising emotion and affect as overlapping. Thus, we use emotion and affect interchangeably in this article to refer to embodied and relational feeling states implicated in what gets included or excluded from MyBackPain. In particular, we draw on three concepts from Ahmed (2014): (1) the *relationality* of emotions; (2) the *impressions* emotions make – their affects; and (3) whether emotions suggest a *directionality* towards or away from particular things.

Relationality – Emotions sit between, link and involve discourse and bodies. They do not (only) sit within humans or non-human objects (or in MyBackPain), but are relational and shifting: '[feelings are] produced as effects of circulation [this] allows us to think of the "sociality" of emotion' (Ahmed, 2014, p. 8). Following critical post-human scholars, the knowing facilitated through the MyBackPain website can similarly be conceptualised as 'embodied, embedded and … flowing in a web of relations' across human and non-humans (Braidotti, 2018, p. 34). Emotions are also discursive, implicated in processes of othering, discipline and conformity (Ahmed, 2010; Ecclestone, 2011). Reflexively attending to our varying affective responses as we journeyed through the website drew our attention to the important nexus between people's lives and discursive elements of MyBackPain. It was impossible, we found, to know the site without considering its relations (affectings/abilities to be affected) with others in the world. To know what MyBackPain *does to the world* (what worlds it makes) was of interest to us, particularly whether it marginalised or excluded any people or ways of being.

Impressions – Emotions are often dismissed in academic health discourses as threats to rational judgement (Damasio, 1994; McNaughton, 2013). However, as Ahmed highlights, emotions are central. People will/do react emotionally when responding to health information. In the case of MyBackPain, we certainly did! We felt comfort, frustration, anger and trust, among other things, and this affected the way we responded to the website's messages. Ahmed (2014, p. 6) might say that the website made an 'impression' on us – in its triple meaning of belief, image or mark. Using Ahmed's concept of impression, we consider how people's emotional relations with MyBackPain can affect the world: they can alter or reinforce beliefs (e.g. how we feel about ourselves); they can change actions (e.g. what treatment choices we make). These emotions make their mark, they impress. Of course, this can go the other way. We too can make an impression on the health messaging and MyBackPain: in how we interpret it and use it; revise it; retell it to others; or craft similar resources in future.

Directionality – Ahmed (2014, p. 8) suggests that emotions involve '(re)actions or relations of "towardness" or "awayness" from any human or non-human object. In the case of our website, an 'object' can be any element of MyBackPain: words and images used to portray health information, types of messages given, the materiality of the device which displays it. Emotions can pull us towards or push us away from these and other objects; directionality suggests possibilities for change (or stasis). Emotions and affect can help to highlight how objects (website elements and materialities) can help to strengthen and build, or potentially prompt destruction. Deleuze (1988, p. 126) discusses affective relations as 'poison or food?' (or both), referring to their decomposing or building capacity. He asks, '[h]ow can a being take another being into its world, but while preserving or respecting the other's own relations and its world?' (Deleuze, 1988, p. 126). This prompts questions such as: How is the website 'food', and/or 'poison'? Can the website, rooted in post-positivist research (which, in its efforts to generalise often lacks consideration of human diversity) enter the world of humans with LBP without marginalising some people, or ways of being, through lack of attention to human difference, complexity, and diversity? In considering these types of questions, we hope to be supra-disciplinary in order to promote ways to bring post-positivist evidence together with socio-political and material conceptualisations of emotion – not to decompose one or the other but to 'form a new, more "extensive" relation' (Deleuze, 1988, p. 126). We strive to 'blur boundaries without burning bridges' (Braidotti, 2011, p. 26) for a 'generative cross-pollination' (Braidotti, 2018, p. 44) as we use Ahmed's work on emotion and affect to rethink habits of presenting health information, to 'feel our way' (Ahmed, 2014, p. 12).

In this article, we treat emotions as central to decision making in health messaging (Lucherini, 2018). To be clear, we are not arguing that emotions should be taken at face value. Rather, we recognise that emotions *do things* in health (Ahmed, 2014; Dragojlovic & Broom, 2018; Olson, Bellocchi, & Dadich, 2020). They can signal a disjuncture in how things are and how they should be. Affective responses can also reinforce established ideas, materialities, assumptions and social structures. Or they can change them; highlighting constrained potentialities and making taken-for-granted assumptions visible creates new possibilities. The emphasis is less on the specific meanings produced with/through a particular subject, and more on affective capacities shaped through engagement with health information.

Post-qualitative inquiry

As mentioned, we used a post-qualitative approach to rethink the evaluation and production of health resources; we bypassed methodological fetishism to apply Ahmed's theory on emotion/affect directly to our main 'data' source: the website. Post-qualitative inquiry prompted consideration of the 'possibilities' of being 'moved to think, feel and know' (Fullagar, 2017, p. 248) the website differently. As part of the broader development of MyBackPain, approved by the human ethics board of The University of Queensland (#2018000064), we used a collaborative and interdisciplinary approach to enhance our supra-disciplinary potential to analyse MyBackPain. This involved a team (all listed authors) of collaborators of different genders and nationalities, from public health, sociology, physiotherapy, psychology, occupational therapy and an 'expert consumer' with complex LBP and graduate training in social theory. Of the eight authors, four were familiar with post-humanism and critical reflexivity; two with critical reflexivity; and the other two were post-positivist researchers.

We used an iterative process to develop analytic insights. First, team members independently engaged with, explored and critically analysed MyBackPain: noting their emotional entanglement with the website, considering its underlying assumptions and their potential unintended consequences. The team members were invited to do this work using any conceptual/theoretical frameworks they had expertise with to inform the analysis, and were also prompted by two readings: one discussing post-qualitative analysis (Fullagar, 2017) and another a critical, discursive exploration of the concept of 'patient-centred care' (Pluut, 2016). The stated intention was not to directly use the readings as theoretical bases for our analysis, but to foster discussion and some common language.

Second, our individual analyses of MyBackPain were discussed during a team analysis session. The session was roughly guided by the following questions:

- What were your reaction/s to MyBackPain? What did you like/not like?
- Did MyBackPain make you think about LBP differently? If so, how?
- What are dominant views/ways of thinking about LBP in general? In what ways does MyBackPain reinforce and/or challenge these views?
- What humans and non-human interactions are involved in MyBackPain?
- Is anyone/anything excluded from/by this website?

The analysis session was audio-recorded and then condensed by the first author into an interim summary, including: (1) key focal areas for investigation, and (2) possible overarching theoretical approaches to inform the post-qualitative methodology. The summary was then shared with all analysts and refined in response to comments. The focus on affect and emotion was chosen by the team as an approach which diverged significantly from the primarily post-positivist underpinnings of the website, thus contributing to the possibilities for a supra-disciplinary critical post-human analysis. The analysis was then iteratively developed between the authors and condensed into this article.

'Afflexive' explorations

We 'afflexively' explore the website and its affects using Ahmed's concepts of *relationality*, *impressions* and *directionality*. The key focal areas developed through our analysis are discussed under three subheadings: 'other(ed) bodies and lives', 'evidence', and 'responsibility'. *Relationality* and *impressions* provoked fairly descriptive discussions, and *directionality* pushed us toward or away various possibilities and abductions. We move on to discuss implications of this in a separate final section: 'Openings'.

Other(ed) bodies and lives

abandonment, exclusion, anger, fear[1]

Ahmed's concept of *relationality* invites a consideration of what MyBackPain does, relationally. The site relates with many human and non-human things, but of particular interest to the health space is how it relates to human lives and bodies (and their health). MyBackPain is explicitly about embodied pain-in-the-low-back situated within lives. We asked, do these relations work well with all lives? Our response: no.

Our analysis of which bodies and lives MyBackPain works for (or not) first arose in relation to pictures of seven people on the homepage. Ostensibly they were images of people with different characteristics – one black woman, three white women, one white man and one First Nations Australian man – all aged between 20 and 50 years. Although these images contributed some visible diversity, there was a subtler level of sameness – all were happy, well-groomed; all appeared to be engaged in 'productive' activities (physical activity and/or paid work); all were thin; all appeared able bodied. The authors involved in producing MyBackPain (Jenny and Paul) discussed how they attempted to source a range of images for the site, but economic constraints and temporal restrictions on negotiations with website developers meant that there were limited possibilities for sourcing/creating images. Jenny and Paul 'chose' to use images produced for mass markets ('stock' images) and available for a small cost but that often exclude most of life's usual messiness, complexities and blemishes. Capital market forces drive the stock image companies' preference for professional models, simple backgrounds and image editing. These intra-actions produce fairly narrow visual representation assemblages within MyBackPain that were reified in the website text. Universal advice (e.g. to keep working and keep active) contained little consideration of the nuances of different lives.

Through 'afflexive' attention to our embodied responses to MyBackPain, many of us noted feelings of exclusion, abandonment, anger for those parts of ourselves and other humans that don't smile, aren't productive, have blemishes. We reflected that some people and lives are more valued than others on the website as we encountered images and words that constrained complexities and reproduced assumed norms. Following Ahmed, we reflected that the MyBackPain assemblage made an 'impression' on us – that only some bodies and lives are valid. Thus, MyBackPain might impress on some users that their bodies and lives are not valid: not neat, orderly and productive lives, able and thin bodies.

This diffuse affective response of exclusion and abandonment suggested *directionality*: MyBackPain might push some people away from the site, even if only temporarily, and draw others in. Consequently, MyBackPain may not enact equitable access to health resources. Although it is a website available at any time, from any location with internet connection, it excludes some people. Noting this directionality usefully indicates a need to consider how to reduce this exclusion while maintaining elements that 'drew people in'.

We did find aspects of MyBackPain which displayed different bodies and lives in its pixels: videos. The production of the videos differed considerably from the stock image assemblages discussed above. They were produced by the industry partner (Arthritis Australia – a consumer advocate organisation), and included researchers, clinicians and experts-through-experience with diverse bodies, ethnicities and relationships to LBP. The lack of a 'studio' setting or 'ideal' environment (particularly for sound) meant that filming was conducted in various environments: around a university, and various healthcare settings. Although not in people's everyday lives, the videos were visibly different to each other and had some ability to attend to the complexities of LBP within different social and material contexts and highlight potentially emotionally challenging and rewarding aspects of living with LBP. The 'more-than-professional' editing meant that nuances were more present, and not edited out. Yet the anticipated bandwidth available (types of wires, internet providers) and typical attention span of website viewers meant that videos were highly edited with some complexities abandoned.

Overall, the website prioritised diverse types of LBP (e.g. short-term, long-term), over diverse social bodies and lives: an unintended outcome. As author Paul (a post-positivist researcher, physiotherapist and one of the creators of the website) said during the analysis session: 'We are giving a really specific message about what is "normal", which I hadn't seen, and that worries me.' Despite its frequent attention to different types of back pain, MyBackPain implicitly assumed all people are the same (or aspire to the same normative ideal – see more on this below in the discussion of 'responsibility'). Thus, the site did not account for the inter-relatedness of these material realities. Taking an afflexive analytic approach highlighted that the website seldom attended to the embodied social and material complexities of accessing the suggested LBP management (e.g. economic, resource or time poverty, experiences of marginalisation) that affect abilities to carry out messages delivered by MyBackPain.

Evidence

frustration, comfort, bewilderment, de-validation (of emotions)

Next, we explore the most heavily referenced section of the website, the 'treatments' section. On this page, approximately 80 different types of treatments for LBP are listed, organised by the website's structured programming (content management system) into numerous subcategories ranging from acupuncture to surgery to exercise. Each treatment is accompanied by an information page, including a rating of the treatment's level of evidence: effective, may be effective, not effective, harmful, lacking evidence. A written description of the treatment and level of evidence was then provided, and pros and cons discussed (largely based on the same evidence). A list of references was provided at the end of each treatment, linking the website with (only positivist) sources.

In its intra-actions with 'the evidence', MyBackPain prioritised positivist evidence: research employing methodologies such as randomised controlled trials, systematic reviews, meta-analyses and case cross-over designs (Eakin, 2016). This prioritisation is unsurprising considering that the site was developed and guided primarily by quantitative/positivist researchers, although at times input from others provided alternative perspectives. The 'post-' part of 'post-positivism' typically came in during an introductory page suggesting that 'no one treatment will work for every person' and 'it is important to think about: which treatments suit your back pain, which treatments suit your beliefs and lifestyle, potential benefits and risks, and possible costs (time, money)'. Beyond these comments, little else guided how treatments might work differently in people's lives.

The treatment section of MyBackPain induced mixed responses amongst us as a research team when considering it 'afflexively'. *Relationally* we felt comfort in having trustworthy research assemblages inform advice about treatment efficacy on the webpage, and relieved that the website did the work for us of gathering and evaluating many forms of treatments. Post-positivist evidence produces legitimacy through statistically-based indications of what works or does not work. And there is some comfort in that. However, this is not the end of the story. Understanding how to integrate this information is important.

Although the tapping of fingers on a screen or a keyboard produced a long list of treatments for eyes (or ears if using a screen reader) and brains to interpret, few of the assembled treatments had evidence to support their effectiveness. Most of us felt frustration that, on the one hand the website suggests that people with LBP can choose what treatment/s they might engage with by listing 80 types of treatments, while on the other hand suggesting that not much 'works'. The post-positivist treatment assemblage produces a need for conclusive evidence, universal approaches, medical cures. We read that 'nothing conclusively 'works' and are frustrated with the failed medical machine rather than reading 'everyone is different and these *might* 'work'' and then feel something else (like hope or curiosity). Although it might be helpful to know that many of the treatments for LBP are unlikely to work, the website does little to attend to the emotional aspects of encountering this information. The website provided 'facts' but not support for how they are received – the restrictions of the website design and responsiveness meant that feelings of frustration cannot be explored in relation in this human-website assemblage – this might be different in other circumstances (for example during a human-human assemblage when someone with LBP asks a friend or a health professional about treatment options).

Even for suggestions supported by post-positivist evidence, there was little guidance regarding how to engage with the sociomaterialities of 'doing' these treatments: engagement remained at the cognitive level. For example, one of the few treatments supported by a high level of evidence was 'keeping active'. Author Kate O'Halloran, who lives with considerable long-term LBP, said:

> I feel unsure about how to proceed with the recommendation that I so often come up against: movement and activity. So often this is suggested and yet for so many in chronic pain this is a source of flare ups, and anxiety about how bad the flare up is. Questions surface: Is this one of those situations where I've crossed the pain threshold without any chance of danger? Or am I still in some kind of danger? My brain oscillates between wondering if I'm 'really [in danger of being] injured' or 'chronically over-sensitised'. For me the website did little to answer those more complex questions which again led to me feeling further frustration.

The website's affective *impressions* are evident here. Frustration (and trust) makes its mark: Kate is left to engage materially (or not) in the suggested 'treatments' without support to negotiate emotional nuances of this engagement.

There are emotional and existential questions incited by MyBackPain, such as: 'Is it normal to be unsure of what to do?' 'Are there ways to integrate or accept uncertainty?' There are material affects of the varied answers to these questions: impressions are made, the body's chemical makeup changes, actions are taken or not taken. The website, as it stands, does little to respond; positivism/quantitative research is ill-suited to these types of enquiries. Yet, other types of 'evidence' were largely excluded from the website assemblage. Our afflexive analysis highlights the website's shortcomings in attending to how the (post-)positivist information might be received and enacted, and in offering other forms of understanding that might be required to engage more flexibly with the social and material complexities of living with LBP.

The *directionality* here suggests there needs to be a reassessment and re-doing of what qualifies as evidence. Post-positivist evidence is valuable when considering which treatments work in controlled circumstances, with some consideration that this varies between contexts. However, the directionality suggested by our afflexive interactions with MyBackPain highlights a need for assembling with 'evidence' beyond that which considers effectiveness. Health information should not become fixated solely on reductive understandings of what works, particularly in complex fields such as pain where the most accurate answer is usually 'we really don't know', 'it depends', or 'a combination of things might work' (Buchbinder, Underwood, Hartvigsen, & Maher, 2020). Other questions need to be asked, such as: What can be done differently so that people live well with conditions with uncertain management strategies? What social, emotional and material conditions work well towards meaningful, enjoyable lives when people have LBP? These types of questions are better suited to other forms of 'evidence' and knowledge.

Although less prominent than the post-positivist evidence, we found some occasions where other forms of knowledge formed part of the MyBackPain assemblage. There were videos of people with LBP which engaged the social and material experiences of living with LBP. For example, Frank (who had been a truck driver) discussed that although his back pain didn't improve, his condition prompted him to retrain and, subsequently, his life became more satisfying. Occasionally, more embodied descriptions were provided of the different treatments, similarly shifting the discussion from generalised effectiveness to the social and material aspects of the treatments, such as 'gentle exercise for people of all abilities' (Tai chi) and 'treatment is often very painful at the time and usually causes increased pain and discomfort for several days to a few weeks after the injection' (prolotherapy). However, these discussions were often limited to physical risks (such as side effects or adverse events) and financial costs.

Health information should attend not only to what works or is effective but how to integrate such messages into lives: how to *do* LBP or LBP management; what it means to live well with LBP. This may mean drawing on multiple types of resources and prioritising supra-disciplinarity.

Responsibility

anger, guilt, shame

Our afflexive exploration of MyBackPain also highlighted issues of responsibility (and the underlying connections between responsibility and power). An inherent complexity of presenting health information for people with LBP is the issue of who is perceived to be responsible for health problems. By their nature, these resources target individual humans rather than workplaces, healthcare institutions, or governments. This is a common way of approaching 'person-centred care': empowering individuals to make decisions about their healthcare and take action (Pluut, 2016). Focusing responsibility on individuals, however, contrasts with understandings of the huge contribution of broader social and material factors (e.g. economic wealth, living conditions, social environment) to ill-health, including LBP (Ferreira et al., 2013; Fu, McNichol, Marczewski, & Closs, 2016; WHO, 2008; Wilkinson & Marmot, 2003). In *relating* to MyBackPain, there were times when we felt anger at this individualisation because it can lead to attention/resources being diverted from affecting these more impactful broader sociomaterialities. This 'empowerment' of individual humans sets the conditions for an individual's efforts to be considered insufficient (by themselves or others) if desired results are not achieved. Blame, shame and guilt are understandable emotional affects – their materiality has various potentialities (e.g. increased cortisol levels, social isolation).

In the discursive materiality of MyBackPain, responsibility is primarily placed on individuals by providing information and choices: 'facts' about LBP, treatments available for LBP, information about health professionals, self-help tips and a 'myth busting' quiz. Aligned with contemporary individualistic (neoliberal) micro- and macro-political discourses, one key implicit message underpinning MyBackPain is that the 'burden of LBP' will improve, if only people choose better. With this comes problems associated with creating responsibility; when things don't work it's perceived to be the individual's fault (Mol, 2008).

The website creates a problem which it then attempts to solve: LBP is something that can be fixed by individuals making choices and taking actions. As author Tim Barlott (an occupational therapist) said:

> The emphasis is on regulation and self-management. It's not about user's everyday life, it's about their pain. So, their pain is the problem and the website is here to solve the pain irrespective of how they want to engage in the world.

MyBackPain positions the problem as pain produced by unhelpful psychological or lifestyle habits (and, less often, as abnormal physiology) and incorrect treatment choices. The solution offered is to easily manage (by) yourself. Consequently, a simple tap of a finger on one of the items on a drop-down menu might produce hope or expectations that LBP may decrease, or become easier to manage. There are no immediate problems when things go to plan. But what happens when the material reality is different? A person might not act on their choices, or what they choose to do might not have the desired effects. A sense of personal failure ensues for not acting and choosing wisely. Guilt and shame are material, they *impress* on bodies and leave marks; 'empowerment' materially affects individuals through its individualisation of responsibility.

The affective *directionality* here is towards reducing the enactment of individualisation and/or differently enacting individualisation. How might a reduction of guilt be produced in (intra-action with) this and other health information websites? Let us examine one example that we introduced earlier: advice to stay active. On the one hand, there is fairly strong (positivist) evidence to suggest that keeping active, including maintaining work or returning to work quickly, is related to better LBP outcomes (Dahm, Brurberg,

Jamtvedt, & Hagen, 2010). On the other hand, making people feel guilty if they cannot (or choose not to) work or otherwise be active is also likely to lead to shame, an associated disengagement with healthcare practices and perhaps resultant marks on bodies (e.g. health problems). Ironically, shame about LBP inaction is likely to lead to further inaction (Bunzli, Smith, Schutze, & O'Sullivan, 2015).

A supra-disciplinary approach here might ask whether it is possible to suggest that people keep active *and* avoid the unintended effects of responsibility and blame? One sociomaterial possibility is to reduce blame by shifting entirely from producing resource assemblages focussed on changing individual behaviour and redirect energies towards social or socio-political change (e.g. addressing the material and social contexts that lead to ill-health, including LBP) – thus shifting the onus for acting away from individuals entirely. For example, material and economic resources could be directed towards re-orienting health services away from reductionist foci towards more broadly conceptualised care for humanity/society. A less dramatic shift might include assembling with socio-material resources that act to reduce the potential shame produced from the individualising messaging on MyBackPain. For example, there could be an engagement with materials that discuss responsibility, shame or guilt as common reactions, and measures to help manage or reduce these effects could be offered.

Openings: what can we do with this?

In response to calls from authors such as Lucherini (2018), we have attended to emotions as an unconventional way to evaluate and rework health resources. We have taken a supra-disciplinary approach, a 'defining feature of the critical posthumanities' (Braidotti, 2018, p. 44), to our afflexive endeavour. In drawing together, relationally and afflexively, embodied and embedded knowing humans with divergent disciplinary perspectives, we have suggested that it is possible to work towards supra-disciplinarity: to achieve a 'shift under multiple pressures' by tapping into our collective 'ability and … willingness to move' and be moved (Braidotti, 2018, p. 44).

By thinking and feeling our way through a worked example using one publicly available health resource, we propose there is much to be gained by taking emotions seriously in health knowledge production/sharing. It helped us imagine how a material resource such as a website might interact with the humans who encounter it. Our afflexive utilisation of Ahmed's conceptualisation of affect and emotion, along with her focus on relationality, impressions and directionality (rather than taking emotions at face-value), provided a way to organise and attend to the complexity and nuance of the website. The approach involves an integration of elements of auto-ethnography (Ellis, Adams, & Bochner, 2011) and critical reflexivity (Kinsella et al., 2012) with affective methodologies and non-representational perspectives.

Afflexivity, as an approach to evaluation, contrasts with conventional rational-cognitive approaches, unconventionally prioritising affective flows. This reworking of evaluation aligns with Kiran, Oudshoorn, and Verbeek (2015) arguments about the limitations of technology evaluations that are only quantitative or 'checklist' in their approach; it suggests that these evaluations are poorly equipped to consider the moral, social and ethical complexities of resources. These 'soft impacts' are critically important: using more social, political and (new) material ways to entangle with the 'object' of our evaluation, such as our afflexive approach, helps to avoid reinforcing or shaping norms in unintended and/or potentially harmful ways (Bjorbækmo & Engebretsen, 2018). Engaging in analyses that can consider such complexities can help avoid inadvertent harms of new health endeavours; this engagement is also likely to encourage adoption (Greenhalgh et al., 2017).

Critical post-humanism is a rapidly developing field (Braidotti, 2018) and we suggest that critically reflexive attention to emotions (afflexivity) is one approach to enacting it. The supra-disciplinary afflexive examination discussed here will help us rework the case study resource (MyBackPain: ArthritisAustralia, 2018). Moreover, our analysis has broader offerings for other health information projects. It poses questions that can be asked of these types of projects such as: How might affect and emotion be consciously considered and fruitfully engaged in a given health resource? In what ways might forms of 'evidence' other than positivist research be utilised in a resource? How might these forms of evidence work *with* positivist research findings to provide a more comprehensive resource for all people? We do not intend to suggest that our approach is the only evaluation that a health resource requires for improvement. However, afflexivity, as we have demonstrated, powerfully enables researchers to explore websites differently, helping to surface issues that might otherwise evade consideration. Our case study offers one such example of engaging with afflexivity to critically evaluate the socio-political, materiality, inclusivity, 'usefulness' and potentialities of an online health resource.

Note

1. There are, of course, many other relevant emotions. This list serves to foreshadow the emotional atmosphere of our analysis.

Disclosure statement

No potential conflict of interest was reported by the author(s).

Funding details

This work was supported by Arthritis Australia's funding; and National Health and Medical Research Council of Australia Fellowships [JS: APP1157199 and PH: APP1102905].

Authorship statement

All authors meet the ICMJE requirements for authorship.

ORCID

Merrill Turpin http://orcid.org/0000-0001-7946-0883
Britta Wigginton http://orcid.org/0000-0001-9265-3583

References

Ahmed, S. (2010). *The promise of happiness*. Durham and London: Duke University Press.

Ahmed, S. (2014). *The cultural politics of emotion* (2nd ed.). Edinburgh: Edinburgh University Press.

Arthritis Australia. (2018). *MyBackPain.org.au*. Retrieved 14th June 2021 from https://mybackpain.org.au/.

Barad, K. (2007). *Meeting the universe halfway: Quantum physics and the entanglement of matter and meaning*. New York: Duke University Press. https://doi.org/10.1215/9780822388128.

Bjorbækmo, W., & Engebretsen, E. (2018). *Clinicians' expectations regarding an e-tablet under development for use in primary care - A critical discussion*. In Sickness and In Health, Sydney, Australia.

Bourdieu, P. (2003). Participant observation: The huxley medical lecture. *Journal of the Royal Anthropological Institute*, *9*(2), 281–294.

Braidotti, R. (2011). *Nomadic subjects: Embodiment and sexual difference in contemporary feminist theory*. New York: Columbia University Press.

Braidotti, R. (2018). A theoretical framework for the critical posthumanities. *Theory, Culture & Society*, 36, 31–61.

Brown, C. A. (2004). The beliefs of people with chronic pain in relation to 'important' treatment components. *European Journal of Pain*, *8*(4), 325–333. doi:10.1016/j.ejpain.2003.10.005

Buchbinder, R., Underwood, M., Hartvigsen, J., & Maher, C. G. (2020). The Lancet Series call to action to reduce low value care for low back pain: An update. *Pain*, *161*(Suppl 1), S57–S64. doi:10.1097/j.pain.0000000000001869

Bunzli, S., Smith, A., Schutze, R., & O'Sullivan, P. (2015). Beliefs underlying pain-related fear and how they evolve: A qualitative investigation in people with chronic back pain and high pain-related fear. *BMJ Open*, *5*(10), e008847. doi:10.1136/bmjopen-2015-008847

Butler, L., & Foster, N. E. (2003). Back pain online: A cross-sectional survey of the quality of web-based information on low back pain. *Spine*, *28*(4), 395–401.

Costa, N., Nielsen, M., Jull, G., Claus, A., & Hodges, P. (2020). Low back pain websites do not meet the needs of consumers: A study of online resources at three-time points. *Health Information Management Journal*, *49*, 137–149.

Cromby, J., & Willis, M. E. H. (2016). Affect or feeling (after leys). *Theory & Psychology*, *26*(4), 476–495. doi:10.1177/0959354316651344

Crotty, M. (1998). *The foundations of social research: Meaning and perspective in the research process*. Sydney: Sage.

Dahm, K., Brurberg, K., Jamtvedt, G., & Hagen, K. (2010). Advice to rest in bed versus advice to stay active for acute low-back pain and sciatica. *Cochrane Database of Systematic Reviews*, *6*, CD007612.

Damasio, A. R. (1994). *Descartes' error: Emotion, reason, and the human brain*. New York: G. P. Putnam's Sons.

Deleuze, G. (1988). *Spinoza: Practical philosophy*. San Francisco: City Light Books.

Deleuze, G., & Guattari, F. (1987). *A thousand plateaus: Capitalism and schizophrenia*. Minesota: University of Minnesota Press.

Dragojlovic, A., & Broom, A. (2018). *Bodies and suffering: Emotions and relations of care*. London: Routledge.

Eakin, J. (2016). Educating critical qualitative health researchers in the land of the randomized controlled trial. *Qualitative Inquiry*, *22*(2), 107–118. doi:10.1177/1077800415617207

Ecclestone, K. (2011). Emotionally-vulnerable subjects and new inequalities: The educational implications of an 'epistemology of the emotions'. *International Studies in Sociology of Education*, *21*(2), 91–113. doi:10.1080/09620214.2011.575100

Ellis, C., Adams, T., & Bochner, P. (2011). Autoethnography: An overview. *Historical Social Research*, *36*(4), 273–290.

Ferreira, P. H., Ferreira, M. L., Maher, C. G., Refshauge, K. M., Latimer, J., & Adams, R. D. (2013). The therapeutic alliance between clinicians and patients predicts outcome in chronic low back pain. *Physical Therapy*, *93*(4), 470–478. doi:10.2522/ptj.20120137

Fu, Y., McNichol, E., Marczewski, K., & Closs, S. J. (2016). Exploring the influence of patient-professional partnerships on the self-management of chronic back pain: A qualitative study. *Pain Management Nursing, 17*(5), 339–349. doi:10.1016/j.pmn.2016.05.004

Fullagar, S. (2017). Post-qualitative inquiry and the new materialist turn: Implications for sport, health and physical culture research. *Qualitative Research in Sport, Exercise and Health, 9*(2), 247–257. doi:10.1080/2159676x.2016.1273896

Gough, B., & McFadden, M. (2013). *Critical social psychology*. (2nd ed). London: Palgrave Macmillan. http://books.google.com.au/books?id=TvqOQgAACAAJ&dq=Gough+and+McFadden&hl=&cd=2&source=gbs_api.

Greenhalgh, T., Wherton, J., Papoutsi, C., Lynch, J., Hughes, G., A'Court, C., … Shaw, S. (2017). Beyond adoption: A new framework for theorizing and evaluating nonadoption, abandonment, and challenges to the scale-up, spread, and sustainability of health and care technologies. *Journal of Medical Internet Research, 19*(11), e367. doi:10.2196/jmir.8775

Haraway, D. (1988). Situated knowledges: The science question in feminism and the privilege of partial perspective. *Feminist Studies, 14*(3), 575–599.

Hendrick, P. A., Ahmed, O. H., Bankier, S. S., Chan, T. J., Crawford, S. A., Ryder, C. R., … Schneiders, A. G. (2012). Acute low back pain information online: An evaluation of quality, content accuracy and readability of related websites. *Manual Therapy, 17*(4), 318–324. doi:10.1016/j.math.2012.02.019

Hodges, P. W., Setchell, J., & Nielsen, M. (2020). An internet-based consumer resource for people with low back pain (MyBackPain): development and evaluation. *JMIR Rehabilitation and Assistive Technologies, 7*(1), e16101. doi:10.2196/16101

Iedema, R., & Carroll, K. (2015). Research as affect-sphere: Towards *spherogenics. Emotion Review, 15*(1), 67–72. doi:10.1177/1754073914544477

Kinsella, E. A., Caty, M., Ng, S., & Jenkins, K. (2012). Reflective practice for allied health: Theory and applications. In E. Kinsella, M. Caty, S. Ng, & K. Jenkins (Eds.), Adult Education and Health. Toronto: University of Toronto Press.

Kiran, A. H., Oudshoorn, N., & Verbeek, P.-P. (2015). Beyond checklists: Toward an ethical-constructive technology assessment. *Journal of Responsible Innovation, 2*(1), 5–19. doi:10.1080/23299460.2014.992769

Laerum, E., Indahl, A., & Skouen, J. S. (2006). What is "the good back-consultation"? A combined qualitative and quantitative study of chronic low back pain patients' interaction with and perceptions of consultations with specialists. *Journal of Rehabilitation Medicine, 38*(4), 255–262. doi:10.1080/16501970600613461

Leys, R. (2017). *The ascent of affect: Geneology and critique*. Chicago: University of Chicago Press.

Lincoln, Y. S., Lynham, S. A., & Guba, E. G. (2013). Paradigmatic controversies, contradictions, and emerging confluences, revisited. In N. K. Denzin, & Y. S. Lincoln (Eds.), *The landscapes of qualitative research* (pp. 199–266). Los Angeles: Sage.

Lucherini, M. (2018). Caught in the middle early career researchers public health and the emotional production of research. *Critical Public Health, 30*. Online first.

Lupton, D. (2020). Vital materialism and the thing-power of lively digital data. In D. Leahy, K. Fitzpatrick, & J. Wright (Eds.), *Social theory and health education: Forging new insights in research*. (pp. 71–80). Milton Park: Routledge.

Massumi, B. (2002). *Parables for the virtual: Movement, affect, sensation*. Durham: Duke University Press.

Maton, K. (2003). Reflexivity, relationism & research: Pierre Bourdieu and the epistemic conditions of social scientific knowledge. *Space and Culture, 6*(1), 52–65. doi:10.1177/1206331202238962

McNaughton, N. (2013). Discourse(s) of emotion within medical education: The ever-present absence. *Medical Education, 47*, 71–79. doi:10.111/j.1365-2923.2012.04329.x

Mol, A. (2008). *The logic of care: Health and the problem of patient choice*. London: Routledge.

Olson, R., Bellocchi, A., & Dadich, A. (2020). A post-paradigmatic approach to analysing emotions in social life. *Emotions & Society, 2*(2), 157–178.

Olson, R., McKenzie, J., & Patulny, R. (2017). The sociology of emotions: A meta-reflexive review of a theoretical tradition in flux. *Journal of Sociology, 53*(4), 800–818. doi:10.1177/1440783317744112

Packer, M. (2011). *The science of qualitative research.* Cambridge: Cambridge University Press.

Pluut, B. (2016). Differences that matter: Developing critical insights into discourses of patient-centredness. *Medicine, Health Care and Philosophy, 19,* 501–515.

Setchell, J., Turpin, M., Costa, N., & Hodges, P. (2020). Web-Based consumer health education about back pain: Findings of potential tensions from a photo-elicitation and observational study. *JMIR Rehabilitation and Assistive Technologies, 7*(1), e17130. doi:10.2196/17130

St. Pierre, E. A. (2021). Post qualitative inquiry, the refusal of method, and the risk of the new. *Qualitative Inquiry, 27*(1), 3–9.

Turner, J. H., & Stets, J. E. (2006). Sociological theories of human emotions. *Annual Review of Sociology, 32,* 25–52. doi:10.1146/annurev.soc.32.061604.123130

Wang, X., Shi, J., & Kong, H. (2020). Online health information seeking: A review and meta-analysis. *Health Communication*, 36, 1–13.

WHO. (2008). World Health Organisation. Closing the gap in a generation: health equity through action on the social determinants of health. Final Report of the Commission on Social Determinants of Health.

Wilkinson, R., & Marmot, M. (2003). *Social determinants of health. The solid facts.* Copenhagen: World Health Organisation.

Index

Note: Figures are indicated by *italics*. Endnotes are indicated by the page number followed by 'n' and the endnote number e.g., 20n1 refers to endnote 1 on page 20.

Abrams, T. 84
Adkins, B. 84
advisory committee for research on women's health (ACRWH) 61
Ahmed, S. 108, 109
Alaimo, S. 2
alcohol and other drug (AOD) scholarship 13
Andaluz, I. 18

Barad, K. 3, 4, 29, 59–61, 91, 93, 100, 102n4, 106
Barlott, T. 105, 115
Berlant, I. 36
Birke, L. 58
blood-borne virus (BBV) 11
Braidotti, R. 106, 107
Bruzzone, S. 2, 90
Butler, J. 14, 29

care for older people (COP): aligning practices 99–100; caring apparatus 92–4; case study 94; digital technologies 90; empirical material, targeting 95–7; homecare 90, 102n3; materialities 91–2; monitoring 97–9; policy strategies 91; political economy 100–2; practices 95
combination therapy 11
Costa, N. 105
COVID-19 public health: drug research 28; health public 37, 38; hotspots 27; intimate counterpublics 37; measures 26; method 30–1; posthumanist performativity 29–30; publics/counterpublics 27; queer counterpublics 35–6; single social bubble 33–5; single-person bubbles 27; stay home, stay safe, analysis 31–3
Cozza, M. 2, 90
Crevani, L. 2, 90

Deleuze, G. 77, 82
direct-acting antivirals (DAAs) 11
domestic and family violence: coercive control 44; COVID-19, coercive control 45–6; ecology 47–8; financial control 44; gendered phenomenon 43; good mother 45; Miranda as method 46–7; social and public health issue 43; women 53
duchenne muscular dystrophy (DMD 79

ecology, domestic violence: home 47–8; money 49–50; pets 52–3; space 50–1; syncretism 48–9; technology 51–2; time 51

Fadyl, J. K. 74
Flore, J. 2, 26
Fraser, N. 30
Fraser, S. 12–14, 20, 21
Fritsch, K. 80
Fujimura, J. 62

Gibson, B. E. 2, 3, 4, 6, 74
Guattari, F. 80

Haraway, D. 58, 106
Hepatitis C 4; AOD scholarship 13, 20; assemblage thinking 13; combination therapy 11; consent/rights 17–19; DAAs 11; drugs 12, 21; policymaking and strategic planning 21; shifting strategies 15–16; testing policies 19; theory/method 13–15; treatment landscape 15; unit of analysis 13; WHO12; opt out approaches 20; novel or innovative strategies 22
Hodges, P. 105
Hörl, E. 47

Kayes, N. M. 74
Kiran, A. H. 116

Law, J. 48, 53
Lawhon, M. 6
Lenton , E. 2, 4, 7, 8, 11

López, A. J. 5
Lucherini, M. 116
Lupton, D. 47

Martiny, K. 85
McCallum, T. 42
Meghji, A. 5
Moore, D. 12–14, 20, 21
Moreton-Robinson, A. 6
Mosleh, D. 74
Murphy, D. 2, 26

O'Halloran, K. 105, 113
Olson, R. 105
online health education: afflexively explore 110–11; directionality 109; directionality: 111; disciplines 107; emotions 108; flattened ontology 106; impressions 108–9; online resources 105; positivism 107; reflexivity 106; relationality 108; scientifically rigorous 106; supra-disciplinary sensibility 107
Oudshoorn, N. 116

Pang, B. 8
Pape, M. 57
Paur, J. 5
person-centred care (PCC): assemblage 76, 77; becoming-chair, experiment 81–2; care-full caring 82–3; caring relationships 82; coda 86; decentred person-care 85–6; evidence-based practice 75; experiment, becoming death life 83–5; humanist case 78; patient voices 74; positivist biomedicine 75; posthuman approach 76; posthuman experimentation 75; posthumanist re-composings 79–81; research case 78–9; respect for persons 74
physiotherapist (PT) 79
Pienaar, K. 2, 8, 26
policy enactments, SABV: data and methods 61–2; material-discursive intervention 60–1; NIH 59
posthuman approaches: Covid-19 public health advice 2; decolonial/feminist/ indigenous scholarship 7; explicit political and ethical frameworks 4–7; feminist posthumanism 4; frameworks 2; health care 2, 3; health practices 1; hepatitis C 4; nonhuman laboratory animals 4; onto-ethical-epistemological assumptions 1; person care 2; posthuman thinking 1; problem 7; public health approaches 8; sociological research 3; socio-material practices 3
post-qualitative inquiry: critical post-humanism 117; evidence 114; health resources 109–10; LBP 112; openings 116–17; relationality 111; responsibility 114–16
Power, J. 2, 26

remade human 2–5 *see also* posthuman approaches
Richardson, S. S. 69
Rock, M. J. 49
Rose, J. 2, 42

science and technology studies (STS) 91
Seear, K. 2, 4, 7, 8, 11
Setchell, J. 2, 6, 105
sex as a biological variable (SABV): animal models *67*; biomedical research 69; feminist biologists 70; gender politics modelling 62–4; gendering laboratory relations 64–6; hormonal/ metabolism-related/morphological traits *63*; NIH policy makers 57, 69; nonhuman agency 58–9; nonhuman entities 58; sex/ restricted integration, gender *64*; varying multiply 66–8
Smith, B. 84
supra-disciplinary approach 116

Terry, G. 74
Thorne Harbour Health (THH) 35
Ticktin, M. 38
Toro, J. 85
Turpin, M. 105

Verbeek, P. -P. 116

Waterworth, K. 74
Wigginton, B. 105

Youdell, D. 43, 47

Zembylas, M. 5